Strategic Thinking

New Frontier for Hospital Management

James B. Webber
and Joseph P. Peters

AHA®

American Hospital Publishing, Inc.,
a wholly owned subsidiary of the
American Hospital Association

Library of Congress Cataloging in Publication Data

Webber, James B.
Strategic thinking.

Reprint. Originally published: Chicago, Ill.: American Hospital Association, c1983.
Includes bibliographical references.
1. Hospitals—Administration. 2. Hospitals—Planning. 3. Corporate planning. I. Peters, Joseph P. II. Title.
RA971.W43 362.1'1'068 84-302
ISBN 0-936450-17-8

Catalog no. 127123

Printed in the U.S.A.
2M-6/83-3-0267
1.5M-2/84-0008
2M-3/85-0080
3.5M-1/86-0133

Tamara Schiller, Editor, Book Division
Marjorie Weissman, Manager, Book Editorial Department
Dorothy Saxner, Vice-President, Books

Contents

List of Figures ... iv

Chapter 1 Introduction ... 1

Part 1 Introduction to Strategic Thinking

Chapter 2 Basic Elements of Strategic Thinking and Management ... 7

Part 2 Analysis and Diagnosis

Chapter 3 Identifying and Evaluating an Institution's Current Strategy ... 21

Chapter 4 Assessing and Monitoring the External Environment ... 27

Chapter 5 Introduction to Forecasting ... 49

Chapter 6 Conducting an Internal Analysis ... 57

Part 3 Strategy Formulation

Chapter 7 Identifying Strategic Alternatives ... 69

Chapter 8 Strategic Choices: Values, Ethics, and Organizational Culture in the Strategic Management Process ... 89

Chapter 9 The Strategic Planning Retreat ... 99

Chapter 10 Preparing for the Future: Real-Life Examples of Formal Strategies ... 107

Chapter 11 From Strategic Thinking to Strategic Management ... 119

Epilogue ... 131

List of Figures

Figure 1 A Strategic Thinking Model 11

Figure 2 Selected Techniques That Link an Organization with Environmental Change 35

Figure 3 Environmental Trend Analysis 36

Figure 4 Stakeholder Analysis 37

Figure 5 How to Do a Simple Competitive Analysis 38

Figure 6 Forces Governing Competition in an Industry 39

Figure 7 Competitive Position Analysis Worksheet 42

Figure 8 Vulnerability Analysis: A Threat Assessment 44

Figure 9 Issues Alert Matrix 45

Figure 10 Internal Areas to Be Analyzed in Assessing Strengths and Weaknesses of a Hospital 59

Figure 11 Range of Strategic Choice: Hospital Strategy 74

Figure 12 Portfolio Analysis 79

Figure 13 The Basic Elements and Relationships in Strategic Planning and Management 123

Figure 14 Three Basic Approaches 128

Chapter 1
Introduction

"Management's job is to control the boundary conditions of the firm, that is, its relationship with its environment."

—C. J. Pearson, *Long Range Planning*[1]

"For the one certainty about the times ahead, the times in which managers will have to work and perform, is that they will be turbulent times. And in turbulent times, the first task of management is to make sure of the institution's capacity for survival, to make sure of its structural strength and soundness, of its capacity to survive a blow, to adapt to sudden change, and to avail itself of new opportunities."

—Peter F. Drucker, *Managing in Turbulent Times*[2]

"Strategy wins wars, wives, elections, business success, and ball games. It determines how the game will be played or the campaign fought. It's intellectual and empirical, theoretical and practical. It motivates commitment and common action. But for many of us, strategy is misunderstood and misused or perhaps even ignored. We might use the word but tack it onto other notions and thereby lose a powerful motive force for achievement."

—William F. Christopher, *Management for the 1980s*[3]

This book is not a text on planning, even though much of its content is essential to good planning. It is basically a how-to-do-it primer on those aspects of hospital management that determine how an institution interacts with its environment. Its goal is to encourage hospital chief executive officers (CEOs) and trustees to think in broader terms than many of them are accustomed: in short, *to think strategically.*

Strategic thinking is a new concept for hospitals. In the past, hospital leaders have devised ways to handle outside forces. However, until recently, with the exception of the 1930s when many institutions were forced to close for economic reasons, most hospital managers have not thought in terms of sheer survival, nor have they been as ruthlessly exposed to such unsettled times. Moreover, hospital CEOs are so pressured by the problems of day-to-day operations that few of them have the time or the inclination to look beyond the moment, even though most of them recognize the importance of planning. Unfortunately, much of hospital planning to date is goal oriented and short range, with heavy emphasis on budgets and facilities or compliance with certificate-of-need requirements. Very few hospital CEOs or trustees practice, much less understand, the corporate strategy concepts described in this book. Perhaps even fewer are aware of the already extensive literature on strategy formulation, strategic management, and long-range forecasting that has emerged from business and industry experiences.

This book is an effort to synthesize these experiences and to show how they can be applied in all types of hospital management settings. Therefore, it is equally useful to large urban medical centers, small rural community hospitals, and voluntary, government, and investor-owned institutions. In addition, everything in this book can be easily implemented by any health care institution whose leaders are committed to good management and to community service.

Thinking strategically adds a new dimension to planning and is best performed as a precursor to the actual planning process. It forces management to look beyond the walls of the institution, to adopt an outside-in view of what is happening. If managers need reminding that many things happening outside are causing problems for hospitals, they need only read the opening pages of Norman McMillan's *Planning for Survival* or almost any issue of *Hospital Week* or other health care periodicals.[4]

Strategic thinking is a vital part of good management; indeed, it is a *sine qua non* of managing a complex enterprise in today's turbulent times. For this reason, strategic thinking is by its very nature a do-it-yourself activity that should not be delegated to an outside party. Unfortunately, not every institution is willing or able to carry out the often very disturbing probings and evaluations that such thinking demands. These institutions have two choices: seek outside help in getting the process started, or take the dangerous risk of doing nothing.

A new strategic model outlined by Merritt L. Kastens best summarizes the many elements of strategic thinking: Here's how we perceive the situation, here's what we believe will happen, here's how we may be affected, and here's what we intend to do about it.[5]

This book is divided into three parts. Part 1 introduces strategic thinking and management by presenting their basic elements. Parts 2 and 3 delineate the two major components of strategic thinking: *analysis and diagnosis* (how we perceive the situation, what we believe will happen, and how we may be affected) and *strategy formulation* (what we intend to do about it). How-to-do-it advice is sprinkled liberally throughout the text for readers eager to get on with the job.

The topics are a distillation of the combined experiences, readings, and reflections of the book's two authors, who have substantial experience in planning and management. James B. Webber began his career in industry, but has recently directed much of his consulting efforts to helping hospitals carry out the processes discussed in this book. He is an independent management consultant and educator specializing in strategic planning for the health care field, with a particular interest in institutional strategy and multi-institutional arrangements among hospitals. However, he has not relinquished his contacts with industry, which is where most of the forward thinking on the subject continues to take place.

Joseph P. Peters has spent his entire career in the health care field, beginning as a hospital administrator and continuing as an areawide health planning agency executive, a part-time lecturer on hospital planning at several major universities, and most recently as an independent consultant in planning for hospitals and health care services.

Do You Have a Strategy?

Before proceeding, readers should ask and honestly answer the following questions, which are specific to the basic matters addressed in the text and provide clues to determining whether the book will be of use to them. More important, the replies will determine whether the reader's hospital is prepared to handle external changes effectively and to meet new needs and the continually heightening expectations of the public it serves.

- Does your hospital have a strategy?
- Are you satisfied with it?
- Are the members of the hospital governing board and top management team aware of the strategy?
- If asked for evidence of this strategy, what types of documents would you present?
- How does the hospital decide which services to offer and what clientele to serve?
- What criteria does the hospital use in making these decisions?
- How does the hospital establish priorities for allocating staff, space, and financial resources?
- How does the hospital evaluate itself to know whether its past strategies have been successful?
- Can you think of any U.S. organizations that have recently changed strategy or direction as a result of changing outside conditions, technological developments, new competition, or changing consumer expectations and needs?
- Can you think of any organizations or firms, including hospitals, that have gone out of business because of any of these changes?
- Do you believe that these questions are of any real value in managing a hospital or in determining your own approach to management?

Definitions

The following key terms will recur throughout the text. Refer to them as often as necessary, because they are essential to the overall process.

1. *Strategy* is a way of thinking when working with change. It is a framework that guides the choices that determine how a hospital interacts with a changing environment. A strategy statement provides both direction and cohesion to the institution's future actions.
2. *Strategic planning* assists management in making nonrecurring, significant decisions that affect the basic nature and direction of the organization. It is a management process that includes periodic strategy formulation, program planning, and operational planning.
3. *Strategy formulation* is the process by which a hospital prepares a statement of direction, taking into consideration changes in the outside world, its resources and values, and the nature and roles of other health care organizations that share its market (its competitors) and a comparable position within the community.
4. *Program planning* uses the strategy statement as a basis for making choices among various program opportunities. Individual programs are evaluated and ranked in terms of the attractiveness of each and the position of the hospital with respect to other institutions offering similar programs. Program planning results in establishing priorities for investment, space, and staffing of future programs. It is often the first step in developing new facilities.
5. *Operational planning* requires middle management and department heads to analyze the planning challenges and issues derived from the strategy formulation and program planning activities and to apply them to their own activities or areas of responsibility. A series of discussions take place between the top hospital management and the department heads. These discussions lead to approved departmental plans, which serve as the basis for resource allocations and future short-term operations. Annual operating budgets are examples of this type of planning.

6. *Strategic issues management* is the continuing capability of identifying and monitoring strategic issues and of managing an institution's response as issues arise. The results of these activities are inputs to periodic strategy formulation.

As Peter Drucker has wryly observed, even good intentions must sooner or later degenerate into work.[6] The time must come to act if strategic thinking is to produce meaningful results; so, too, the time has come to close this introduction and to urge readers to move into the text itself.

Notes

1. Pearson, C. J. Setting corporate objectives as a basis for action. *Long Range Planning.* 12:15, Aug. 1979.
2. Drucker, Peter F. *Managing in Turbulent Times.* New York City: Harper & Row, Publishers, 1980, p. 1.
3. Christopher, William F. *Management for the 1980s.* Englewood Cliffs, NJ: Prentice-Hall, Inc., 1980, p. 69.
4. McMillan, Norman H. *Planning for Survival: A Handbook for Hospital Trustees.* Chicago: American Hospital Association, 1978.
5. Adapted from a model in Kastens, Merritt L. Chicken and egg: management and planning. *Planning Review.* 8:10, May 1980.
6. Drucker, Peter F. *Management: Tasks—Responsibilities—Practices.* New York City: Harper & Row, Publishers, Inc., 1974, p. 128.

Part 1

Introduction to Strategic Thinking

Chapter 2

Basic Elements of Strategic Thinking and Management

"Continuous monitoring . . . of the quality and continued suitability of corporate purpose is over time the most sophisticated and essential of all the functions of management. . . The perspective which sustains this function is the kind of creative discontent which prevents complacency even in good times and seeks continuous advancement of corporate and individual capacity and performance. It also requires constant attention to the future, as if the present did not offer problems and opportunities enough."

—Kenneth R. Andrews, *The Concept of Corporate Strategy*[1]

"In business as on the battlefield, the object of strategy is to bring about the conditions most favorable to one's own side, judging precisely the right moment to attack or withdraw and always assessing the limits of compromise correctly. Besides the habit of analysis, what marks the mind of the strategist is an intellectual elasticity or flexibility that enables him to come up with realistic responses to changing situations, not simply to discriminate with great precision among different shades of gray."

—Kenichi Ohmae, *The Mind of the Strategist: The Art of Japanese Business*[2]

"[S]trategic thinking is a logical exploration and retrieval process, not a mechanistic set of norms or ideas. It is based on disciplined questioning and recording, not on any magic formula that will supply revelations and somehow guarantee success for the user who goes through the ritual."

—William E. Rothschild, *Putting It All Together: A Guide to Strategic Thinking*[3]

Hospitals are complex organizations that are difficult to manage even in the best of times. As with any corporate enterprise, hospitals operate in a dual environment of time and place filled with uncertainties of change over which they have little or no control. Moreover, the nature of their work and clientele make hospitals more susceptible to external change than most other enterprises.

When times are turbulent, hospital management faces the added difficulty of confronting sudden, often erratic situations that can threaten the survival of the institution or affect its activities in unexpected ways. But turbulence not only presents threats and risks to an organization, it also offers opportunities and challenges. A major task of top management is to identify these important problems, issues, and opportunities that develop in the environment and to devise appropriate ways of handling them. The process of carrying out this task is called strategic management, and the result is known as the organization's *strategy*.

Strategy is a favorite word in management lexicon. As a noun, it summarizes the nature and direction of an organization in interacting with its environment or it can be used in a more general sense to indicate that an organization knows what it wants to do and how to do it. In its adjectival form, it modifies many terms associated with the overall management or decision-making function, for example, strategic planning, strategic alternatives, strategic choice, strategic thinking, strategic funds programming, and strategic business units.

Many definitions of strategy have been advanced by knowledgeable authors and practitioners in many fields of human endeavor. All bear a resemblance to the original military use of the term, which involves accepting an existing situation or anticipating a future situation and adapting to it. All of the definitions incorporate a future time dimension, a conscious purpose, and a sense of direction, which are summarized in a statement capable of being communicated to those affected by or expected to carry out the strategy.

Some Contemporary Definitions of Strategy

"Strategy denotes general attention to the basic means for the conduct of war, its duration, its intensity, and its geographic scope. It examines the means and methods of preparing the armed services for war while taking into account political requirements, economic potential, scientific and technical accomplishments, and various other factors pertaining to the organizational and resource capabilities of its armed services to solve strategic problems. Strategy is, therefore, the leading element, because it determines the general aim, the forces employed, and the methods used to solve the relevant problems."

—Marshal V. D. Sokolovsky,
Military Strategy: Soviet Doctrine and Concepts[4]

"Strategy is a focused concept for development of the business—a statement of product and market commitments, with implications for technology, structure, and operations.

"Successful managing requires a concept of the business: active exploration of opportunities and challenges in the environment and explicit choices about what the business should become."

—Igor H. Ansoff, *Corporate Strategy: An Analytic Approach to Business Policy for Growth and Expansion*[5]

"Corporate strategy is the pattern of major objectives, purposes, or goals and essential policies and plans for achieving those goals, stated in such a way as to define what business the company is in or is to be in and the kind of company it is or is to be.

"Strategy formulation has to do with the reconciliation of conflicting answers to these questions:
- What might we do (in terms of environmental opportunity)?
- What can we do (in terms of ability and power)?
- What do we want to do (in terms of personal preferences)?
- What should we do (in terms of social responsibility)?"

—Kenneth R. Andrews, *The Concept of Corporate Strategy*[6]

"Corporate strategy can best be defined by looking at the purposes it serves: to provide both direction and cohesion to the enterprise. Providing direction is the traditional objective assigned to corporate strategy: to give the company a sense of purpose and mission. Providing cohesion, on the other hand, is an objective of corporate strategy which is often ignored. Yet it is not only important but also more essential than providing direction."
—Hugo Uyterhoeven and others, *Strategy and Organization: Text and Cases in General Management*[7]

"An organization's strategy is a statement of the fundamental means it will use, subject to a set of environmental constraints to try to achieve its objectives. Alternately, an organization's strategy is the fundamental pattern of present and planned resource deployments and environmental interactions that indicates how the organization will achieve its objectives."
—Charles W. Hofer and Dan Schendel, *Strategy Formulation: Analytical Concepts*[8]

"Strategy is a framework which guides those choices that determine the nature and direction of the organization."
—Benjamin B. Tregoe and John W. Zimmerman, *Top Management Strategy, What It Is and How To Make It Work*[9]

"A strategy is a unified, comprehensive, and integrated plan relating the strategic advantages of the firm to the challenges of its environment. It is designed to ensure that the basic objectives of the enterprise are achieved."
—William F. Glueck, *Strategic Management and Business Policy*[10]

As used in this book, strategy is simply a way of thinking when dealing with change. It is a framework that guides the choices about how an organization—in this instance, a hospital—will interact with a changing world. A statement of strategy provides both direction and cohesion to the institution.

Every organization or its leadership has some sort of strategy, however vague, that directs the nature of its operations and sets its goals. It may exist only in the mind of one person or it may reflect the shared experiences of top management. In some instances, it may be so outdated that it gives little direction to the organization or cannot unify the various activities of the enterprise into a cohesive whole. In other instances, it may be built on a systematic and disciplined strategic thinking process that continually attempts to match the organization's competencies and resources with the opportunities and challenges of its environment.

Most hospital strategies and, indeed, the strategies of most corporate enterprises fall somewhere between these two extremes. Most strategies are incremental in nature and unplanned in practice, based more on off-the-cuff pronouncements than on a formal strategic thinking effort. Rarely are they expressed in a written form that can be communicated to others within or outside the organization.

This is so because hospitals originate from a long tradition of humanitarian concerns and charitable impulses. They are, in a real sense, single-purpose enterprises organized to fulfill the needs of the sick and injured, although many hospitals have since expanded their efforts to a variety of related activities. The need for their services has been so clear-cut that few of them have found it necessary to prepare anything more than a legal statement of corporate purpose.

Perhaps the reason most hospitals fail to think in strategic terms exists in the nature of their management. More than 90 percent of United States' hospitals are governed by appointed or elected boards, commissions, or overseers who are neither employed by the institution nor, with some exceptions, associated with its medical staff. The members of these governing bodies traditionally have been accountable mainly to themselves or to those who appointed them. Their concerns have been directed more toward obtaining and conserving their institutions' resources than monitoring the institutions' ability to adapt to the demands of a complex and dynamic environment.

Signs indicate that this may be changing. The recent emphasis on long-range planning has led many hospitals to ask probing questions about the reasons for existence, the needs of their communities, and the nature of their competition, and many have taken the added step of writing more meaningful mission statements.[11] Some hospitals are now employing marketing concepts and techniques to think systematically about their relationships with the outside world and their clientele.[12] Other hospitals are adapting corporate models to their organization and management. This move to corporate models may lead to a greater awareness of the importance of strategic thinking in the management of hospitals. However, despite the increased use of these new ideas, the institution that is prepared or willing to engage in the type of strategic thinking that constitutes the theme of this book is still the exception.[13]

Strategic Thinking in a Nutshell: One Expert's View

"The strategic thinking process begins with the most important component of your organization's life: you. What is the nature of your business, and what does it want to become? The next analysis concentrates on the source of your business existence, namely, your customers. Evaluations of your industry and markets emerge from your exploration of 'the game" you're in, and you turn next to a detailed assessment of your most important fellow players—your key competitors. Equipped with such insights about the external world, you can then evaluate your own organization's capabilities. These analyses make it possible for you to choose the kind of strategy you wish to pursue. Ultimately, they provide an estimation of the risks, costs, and rewards you can expect and a determination of the objectives you can realistically achieve."

—William E. Rothschild, *Putting It All Together: A Guide to Strategic Thinking*[14]

As quasi-public enterprises, hospitals are under pressure from many external groups: the public clamors for hospitals to be more accountable to consumers, legislators devise various regulatory schemes to control rising costs of health care, planning agencies seek to influence the development and distribution of hospital resources, health insurers worry about overuse of inpatient services, manufacturers entice hospitals with new technologies and products unheard of a decade ago, labor unions vie to represent workers who have traditionally been at the low end of the wage spectrum, and licensing and accrediting bodies tighten what are already strict standards. In addition to all of these group interests and pressures are the broader forces of social, demographic, economic, and political change that have an impact on what hospitals do, whom they serve, and how they are financed and managed.[15] Strategy provides not only a sense of direction in meeting these external challenges and demands, but it also supplies the lead time to ponder the implications of these pressures on the future of the institution.

What is the strategic thinking process that hospitals are being urged to incorporate into their management techniques? How does it differ from the long-range planning activities in which many hospitals are already engaged? Who develops an institution's strategy? Is the resulting strategy statement simply a synonym for a mission statement? What are the thought processes and logic that form the basis for developing an effective strategy? Although the answers to these questions are not in a strict sense how-to-do-it matters, they are important to an understanding of strategy and how it can be applied to hospital management situations.

Strategic Thinking Model

Strategic thinking is simply a variation of a well-known, four-element approach to problem solving: problem finding, problem definition, problem solving, and implementation of the problem solution. The basic strategic thinking model translates and expands the four elements into the following sequence of steps (see figure 1, A Strategic Thinking Model):

- Searching the environment to determine those forces or changes that may affect the work of the organization or that may be crucial to its survival
- Appraising the organization's strengths and weaknesses—its potential for dealing with change
- Identifying the major strategic opportunities and threats

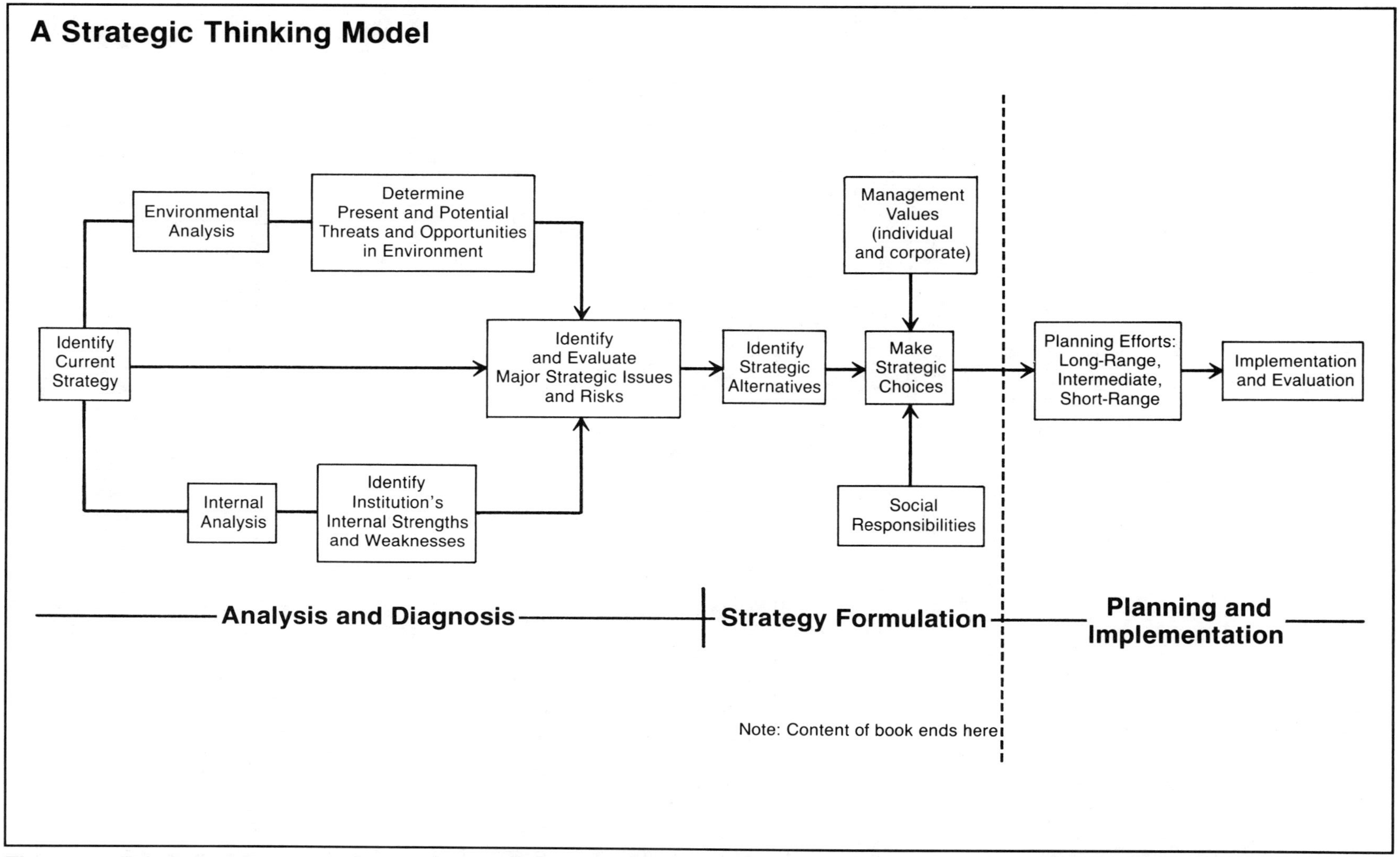

Figure 1. This model translates the elements of problem solving into a sequence of steps. These steps should be tailored, as necessary, to the needs of the specific organization.[16]

- Identifying and evaluating the various strategic options available to the organization in meeting these opportunities and threats
- Selecting the option that best balances the organization's potential with the challenges of changing conditions, taking into account the values of its management and its social responsibilities
- Preparing the strategy
- Implementing and evaluating the strategy

Neither this nor any other strategic model can be applied indiscriminately to all situations. The various tasks should be tailored to the specific needs and complexities of the organization and to the interests and backgrounds of its leaders. In fact, as the participants gain experience in carrying out the process, both the model itself and the component tasks can be revised or modified. As has been wisely stated, "What counts in the end is the quality of the analysis and the soundness of the final strategy, and not the elegance of the process or system that produces the strategy."[17] And the following piece of advice is always appropriate and important to such a task: *keep it simple.*

Strategic Thinking and Planning

A distinction between strategic thinking and planning must be made, because many managers use the two terms interchangeably. This is understandable in light of the growing popularity of strategic planning in management circles. However, not only are there important conceptual differences between strategic thinking and planning, but paradoxically, planning can be a deterrent to strategic thinking.[18]

As already noted, strategic thinking helps an organization determine the direction in which it should move in its passage through the time and place of its environment. By its very nature, strategic thinking is adaptive, responsive, and fraught with risk because its focus is always on the environment. More important, strategic thinking helps mold the "personality" or image of the enterprise by spelling out what Benjamin B. Tregoe calls the *driving force* of the organization's efforts.[19] Although hospitals have many similar goals and programs, noticeable differences in the personalities of institutions exist. Some hospitals exemplify aggressive growth and diversification. They seem always ready to explore new opportunities, to commit themselves to new ventures, to establish outreach programs, to add more beds and services, or to dominate their local medical markets. These institutions have an obvious growth strategy, even though it may not be formally written down. Other institutions seem content to be more selective in their activities. They are rarely pacesetters, but are willing to add new programs and services when these seem necessary to keep abreast of competition. Their strategies are basically defensive and imitative.

Some institutions show little interest in change. They act as if traditional ways of managing their affairs need not be altered. They are usually more interested in defending the past than in exploring the future. Many of them display little interest in looking beyond their walls, with the result that they rarely offer outreach services, wellness programs, or any of the new community health services that are being emphasized. If they have an expressed strategy, it is apt to be couched in such self-laudatory, flowery claims as "supplying warm, personalized services" in a "friendly, patient-centered environment" or other clichés that offer no direction for the future. Recent events have harshly affected some of these hospitals, often forcing them to merge with more strategically minded institutions or to cease operation entirely.

Planning is *operations-oriented* and focuses primarily on the setting of goals and how to achieve them; hence, its great emphasis on management by objectives. Much of hospital planning is necessarily short range in outlook, and even long-range plans may specify immediate actions as first steps in moving toward more distant goals. However, this necessity does not diminish the need for or lessen the importance of planning. *It simply indicates that something more basic must precede planning: that something is strategy.*

Good planning rests on good strategy and, indeed, a good strategy shapes the plan. An organization should know in *what* direction it wishes to move before determining *how* to get there. Many hospitals confuse the two dimensions. Therefore, they move too quickly into the planning stage and either ignore or rush through the analyses that form the basis for the strategic thinking phase.

Some Basic Approaches to the Logic of Strategy

Traditional Approach to Hospital Planning

Mission ⟶ Goals ⟶ Priorities ⟶ Objectives ⟶ Actions

Much of hospital planning in the past has involved the preparation of a mission statement that, in turn, is translated into goals and objectives that can be achieved in a specified time frame by the institution's various operating entities.[20]

Gap-Bridging Approach

Goals ⟶ Analyses ⟶ Gaps ⟶ Options ⟶ Choice ⟶ Actions

Gap-bridging is a variation of the traditional approach. Its logic is straightforward: an institution selects appropriate actions to bridge the gap between its present positions (where it is) and a desired future position (where it would like to be).[21]

Issue-Oriented Strategic Thinking

External Analysis ⟶ Internal Analysis ⟶ Issues ⟶
Alternatives ⟶ Choice ⟶ Plan ⟶ Actions

This approach is the preferred option outlined in this book. It focuses on identifying significant issues that signal the need for a possible change in direction that must be addressed by a hospital as it anticipates changes in its internal and external environments.

Strategic Updating or Evaluative Approach

Current Strategy ⟶ Analyses ⟶ New Future Strategy ⟶
Plan ⟶ Actions

This approach presupposes that a hospital has a defined strategy that can be examined in light of new developments and, if necessary, updated to accommodate anticipated emerging opportunities, challenges, and threats. As hospitals gain experience in thinking strategically, much of their future strategic management efforts will center on this approach.

Strategists

Who creates an organization's strategy? Experts agree—and experience in all types of enterprises supports their view—that this is the job of top management. Not only are the top managers personally responsible for preparing strategy, but they are also equally responsible for making the strategy work.

Experience indicates that an organization should mobilize its 12 best thinkers for this task. To be sure, entrepreneurial managers have often been able to catapult their firms to prominent positions through their own efforts or by forcing their views on the rest of management. However, successful managers now also realize that strategy is the province of more than one person, a select group of individuals. In fact, it is not even necessary to follow organizational lines to constitute this group. The major qualifications are a working knowledge of the organization and the intellectual ability to carry out the strategic thinking process.

Here lies a basic difference between strategy formulation and long-range planning. Long-range planning is best accomplished by a more representative, and often larger, group of individuals from within and outside of the organization who meet on a continuing, regular basis to carry out the various planning tasks. The strategists are a more select group that meets only when necessary, perhaps only a few times, to formulate the overall direction of the subsequent planning efforts.

Hospitals face special problems in constituting this group. Although hospitals, with few exceptions, are not large compared with many businesses, their organizational structure and administrative arrangements are more complex and more rooted in tradition. The top-level triad of governing board, administration, and medical staff is unique, and the interrelationships are often knotty and sometimes adversarial. If a hospital develops a strategy, it must somehow emerge from this top-level organizational triad. If the strategy is to work, it must also have the support of the three groups or, at least, none should oppose or in other ways undermine it.

A hospital must also be prepared to balance and negotiate with many other groups that contribute to its work or that are affected by its programs. These include its patients, other individuals in its local community or market who are prospective recipients of its services, employees, volunteers and auxilians, suppliers and creditors, philanthropic donors, government officials at all levels, health insurers, professional associations, labor unions, and health planning bodies. Of course, representation from all of these parties in an institution's strategic management process is neither feasible nor practical. However, wise management is alert to the needs, demands, and expectations of these constituencies and usually finds ways to incorporate these outside interests into its decision-making efforts.

In most hospitals, the governing board has the responsibility for ensuring that the institution has a strategy for encountering the future. However, most trustees or directors do not know the organization well enough to carry out a strategic management process alone. Some of them should participate in the process, but these persons must be carefully selected in accordance with their ability to contribute significantly to the process. Nevertheless, *a major responsibility of the board of any organization is to review and ratify strategy proposals prepared by the 12 best thinkers and, over time, to evaluate the effectiveness of the strategy to ensure the purposeful development of the enterprise.*[22]

Role of the CEO

> "Probably the skill most nearly unique to general management, as opposed to the management of functional or technical specialties, is the intellectual capacity to conceptualize corporate purpose and the dramatic skill to invest it with some degree of magnetism. No sooner is a distinctive set of corporate objectives vividly delineated than the temptation to go beyond it sets in. Under some circumstances it is the chief executive's function to defend properly focused purpose against superficially attractive diversification or corporate growth that glitters like fool's gold. Because defense of proper strategy can be interpreted as mindless conservatism, wholly appropriate defense of a still valid strategy requires courage, supported by detailed documentation."
>
> —Kenneth R. Andrews, *The Concept of Corporate Strategy*[23]

CEOs of large hospitals tend to exercise more influence in the development of strategy than do their counterparts in small institutions. Large hospitals are better able to recruit seasoned administrators and to supply them with necessary operating and staff support to perform their management responsibilities. Large hospitals have also been among the first to incorporate planning into their overall management process. A recent study has indicated, moreover, that CEOs of large hospitals have more leeway in the strategic planning process and that administrators of small rural hospitals are often obliged to seek approval from their medical staffs and other interested parties in implementing strategic change.[24] The highly developed strategies of some large market-oriented hospitals with highly diversified programs are often the efforts of skillful CEOs who are clearly the "architects of purpose" for their institutions.[25]

Consultants can play an important role in assisting hospitals in their strategic management and planning activities. However, given the nature of strategic management, one can properly ask when and why an institution should turn to an outside consultant for help. Indeed, a key question is not whether consultants can be helpful—simply too much evidence exists to indicate that they can be—but rather, do some hospitals rely too heavily on consultants by asking them to do what the institutions can or should be able to do themselves?

The dilemma of relying on outside help versus doing it yourself is not easy to resolve. As one consultant recently observed, "A consultant can do nothing that the hospital couldn't do if the hospital had the staff, the time, and the objectivity."[26] Unfortunately, many hospitals have neither the staff, the time, nor the objectivity to pursue a well-conceived strategic management effort without some outside assistance. Therefore, it may be more appropriate to ask what should be expected of consultants. Should they actually devise a strategy for an institution and submit it to the governing body for approval? Should they simply serve as catalysts by getting the process under way (conducting a retreat for the board and top management is an increasingly popular first step)? Should they be asked to perform various studies and assessments, such as those discussed later in this book? Should they be viewed basically as experts in making strategic choices? Or, should they intervene in other ways and, if so, how? Again, there are no easy answers to these questions. Consultants can and often are asked to do any or all of these tasks.

At best, perhaps the only recommendation that can be made about the use of consultants is as follows: *Employ consultants to do what the institution cannot otherwise do for itself because of a lack of in-house capabilities; but do not ask them to do anything that, according to rules of good management, the organization should do for itself.*

In-house staff planners can contribute to various aspects of the strategic management process. Indeed, in many large hospitals (usually with 200 or more beds), these staff members are regarded as in-house consultants by the CEO and by the strategic planning committee. As with outside consultants, in-house planners must be properly utilized and not asked to perform functions that might usurp the responsibilities of top management.

Staff Planners and Strategic Management

"Corporate planners are staff specialists who are trained in the skills of strategic management techniques and who provide staff support services and recommendations on strategic management decisions. Such a staff can participate in many aspects of the strategic management process: it can perform environmental analyses and diagnostic studies, it can study the firm to assess its strengths and weaknesses, it can generate some strategic alternatives and research their feasibility, and it can aid in implementing the strategy chosen in organization and policies. . . . *But all the evidence indicates that such a staff rarely, if ever, seriously participates in the strategic choice process.* This is the crucial job of the top executive, and the staff serves as the executive's research and follow-through team."

—William F. Glueck, *Strategic Management and Business Policy*[27]

An important factor in preparing strategies for hospitals is whether they are organized with major subunits or program areas, termed *strategic business units (SBUs)*. SBUs are operating divisions in a firm that produce distinct products, serve special market segments, or cater to well-defined sets of customers. SBUs are often given the authority to make their own strategic decisions within overall corporate guidelines.[28] Hospital examples include ambulatory care departments, long-term care units, research institutes, satellite and outreach operations, leased hospitals, management agreements, and various shared service and hospital system arrangements.

Not only may individual strategies be needed for these corporate elements, but also the impact of the organization's overall strategy on each of these units must be assessed.[29] If a hospital is organized into SBUs, the heads of these units should be engaged in preparing strategies for their units as well as in the overall strategic management of the organization. How well this is done will, in part, be determined by the abilities and personalities of the unit managers involved and, in part, will reflect the overall style of the hospital's management.

Mission Statement and Strategy

Sooner or later, every organization must face up to the task of defining its basic purposes and mission. It must develop a sense of identity. As Peter Drucker has so wisely stated, "Nothing may seem simpler or more obvious . . . [and yet] 'What is our business?' is almost always a difficult question and the right answer is usually anything but obvious."[30] Indeed, unless management knows what its business is, what its business should be, and what its business will be, it is really not prepared to interact effectively with its environment. Nor will it be able to find a focus for its future efforts. Because a good mission statement can endow everyone in an organization with a vision of something strongly desired, it often provides the cohesiveness and the ability to plan in an integrated fashion that is so essential to designing an organization's future.[31]

The development of a mission is obviously related to strategy, but a mission statement is not a synonym for strategy. It can be either a starting point for the formulation of a strategy or an outcome of the strategic management process. Some situations require that defining the mission precede the development of the strategy, just as the strategy precedes its long-range planning and implementation efforts. The mission is then used to guide the choice of the strategic alternatives. This approach works well when an organization has more control of its destiny than is now possible in such a highly regulated and turbulent environment. These factors often require that a hospital examine and redefine its mission and role as a key effort in its strategic management process. Thus, mission and strategy become part of the same overall process. This is the preferred approach and is treated as such in this book.

Process of Strategic Thinking

Basically, a well-organized strategic management effort involves what George Steiner has described as "an integrated set of institutional arrangements within which decision making can proceed in an orderly fashion."[32] Strategic management and the strategic thinking that supports it are simply variations of the basic decision-making process that constitutes good management. Decisions involve goals to be accomplished and the means to reach them. However, decision making gives answers that, as Benjamin B. Tregoe stresses, "cannot be verified because the actions will take place in the always uncertain future."[33] These actions in the always uncertain future are the concerns of strategy and planning.

A good decision implies that the decision maker has selected the means or option best suited to achieve the desired ends, not by off-the-cuff remarks, emotional choices, or chance selection, but through thoughtful analysis of available information, reasonable conclusions, and appropriate actions—in short, by intelligent, organized thought. Indeed, some observers maintain that the major contribution of the strategic management process and the planning process that results from it is the rationality that they impose on an organization's efforts to anticipate its future.

What is considered rational or its converse, irrational, too often depends on who is making the judgment. Few decision makers can completely remove themselves from their biases or personal frames of reference. What they know and how they know it colors all of their actions and shapes the way in which they contend with the outside world and the problems it presents them. Rationality implies that appropriate alternatives are being considered, that the best available alternative will be selected to achieve the goals or solve the problems, and that the right kind of information and skills will be used judiciously on the matters at hand. Asking the right questions can, at times, be more important than finding the right answers. So, too, is the ability to question the assumptions, values, and biases that underlie forecasts of the future, establishment of goals, strategic choices, and recommended actions.

Problem Structuring and Strategic Thinking

"The kinds of situations that call for strategic thinking are termed ill-structured. They are characterized by difficulty, ambiguity, and the lack of established methods for moving towards clarification. . . . [T]he primary task when facing an ill-structured problem is to reduce ambiguity by structuring the problem. Thus, for our purposes, strategy-making is a response that does not necessarily 'solve' the problem, but which redefines it in terms of more familiar subproblems. . . . Unlike rational-analytic problem solving, the function of strategy is not to 'solve' a problem, but to so structure a situation that the emergent problems are solvable."

—Richard P. Rumelt, *Strategic Management: A New View of Business Policy and Planning*[34]

There is a thought process that hospital management can follow in making rational choices that match the institution's resources and capabilities with the changing requirements of the environment in which it operates. Kenneth R. Andrews summarizes this intellectual process as "ascertaining what a company *might do* in terms of environmental opportunity, of deciding what it *can do* in terms of ability and power, and of bringing these two considerations together in optimal equilibrium."[35] Personal values, ethics, norms, ideals, emotions, and aspirations often influence these decisions by incorporating preferential (what we *want to do*) and normative (what we *should do*) dimensions into the process. In many instances, these nonrational elements do more to shape the strategic outcome than do the thought patterns that underlie the process.

Despite the emphasis on rational choices, strategic thinking is loaded with intuitive choices. Bruce

D. Henderson, a knowledgeable consultant, has noted that "the final choice in all business decisions is, of course, intuitive. It must be. Otherwise, it is not a decision, just a conclusion—a printout."[36]

Recognizing these nonrational elements should not, however, discourage would-be strategists. Strategy making is not a science, nor does anyone seriously expect it to be so. Too many variables, too many differences in form and content of institutional programs and in organizational structure, and too many shadings in abilities, values, and expectations of the participants exist to allow a uniform magic-formula technique appropriate to all institutions. Thus, with some uncommon exceptions, conscious strategy emerges from an intellectual discipline that blends rationality, creativity, intuition, experience, and value judgments into an organized sequential process of analysis, assessment, and choice that matches an organization to its environment. Subsequent chapters describe the various tasks in carrying out this process.

Notes

1. Andrews, Kenneth R. *The Concept of Corporate Strategy.* Homewood, IL: Richard D. Irwin, Inc., 1980, pp. 13-14.
2. Ohmae, Kenichi. *The Mind of the Strategist: The Art of Japanese Business.* New York City: McGraw-Hill, 1982, p. 3.
3. Rothschild, William E. *Putting It All Together: A Guide to Strategic Thinking.* New York City: AMACOM, 1976, p. v.
4. Sokolovsky, Marshal V. D. *Military Strategy: Soviet Doctrine and Concepts.* New York City: Praeger, 1963.
5. Ansoff, H. Igor. *Corporate Strategy: An Analytic Approach to Business Policy for Growth and Expansion.* New York City: McGraw-Hill, 1965.
6. Andrews.
7. Uyterhoven, Hugo, and others. *Strategy and Organization: Test Cases in General Management.* Homewood, IL: Down Jones-Irwin, 1977.
8. Hofer, Charles W., and Schendel, Dan. *Strategy Formulation: Analytical Concepts.* St. Paul, MN: West Publishing Co., 1978.
9. Tregoe, Benjamin B., and Zimmerman, John W. *Top Management Strategy, What It Is and How to Make It Work. New York City: Simon & Schuster, 1980.*
10. Glueck, William F. *Strategic Management and Business Policy.* New York City: McGraw-Hill, 1980.
11. For a list of the types of questions useful in preparing a mission statement, see Peters, Joseph P. *A Guide to Strategic Planning for Hospitals.* Chicago: American Hospital Association, 1979, pp. 64-67.
12. For example, see MacStravic, Robin E. *Marketing Health Care.* Germantown, MD: Aspen Systems Corporation, 1977; MacStravic, Robin E. *Marketing by Objectives for Hospitals.* Germantown, MD: Aspen Systems Corporation, 1980; and Tucker, Stephen L. Introducing marketing as a planning and management tool. *Hospital and Health Services Administration.* 22:37, Winter 1977.
13. In a recent study of 15 Missouri community general hospitals, Douglas C. Mankin and William F. Glueck found little evidence that hospitals in the sample were formally planning their strategies. They noted that "the larger hospitals did a better job in standardizing the process, but this seemed to be more form than substance. Few did an effective job in appraising the environment to anticipate major changes or opportunities." Their findings are reported in Mankin, Douglas C., and Glueck, William F. Strategic planning. *Hospital and Health Services Administration.* 22:6, Spring 1977. In addition, a study of 10 large urban teaching hospitals disclosed that "none of the institutions surveyed felt satisfied with their current planning strategies." See Bander, Kay W. Strategic planning: reality versus literature. *Hospital and Health Services Administration.* Special Issue I. 25:7, 1980.
14. Rothschild, pp. 3-4.
15. For a fuller treatment of the problems and issues facing hospitals, see American Hospital Association. *Hospitals in the 1980s: Nine Views.* Chicago: AHA, 1977, and *Environmental Assessment of the Hospital Industry 1979.* Chicago: AHA, 1979.
16. Based on ideas from Andrews; Glueck; and Hofer and Schendel.
17. Hofer and Schendel, p. 67.

18. Most of the ideas discussed in this section are derived from Tregoe, Benjamin B., and Zimmerman, John W. Strategic thinking: key to corporate survival. *Management Review.* 68:8, Feb. 1979. Those interested in pursuing the relationship of strategic thinking to planning and in obtaining a deeper understanding of why the former must precede the latter will gain much from this article. See also Tregoe, Benjamin B., and Zimmerman, John W. Don't jump too quickly into goal-setting. *Industry Week.* 180:48, Feb. 11, 1974; and Rothschild, 1976.

19. Tregoe and Zimmerman, 1979, p. 9.

20. See, for example, Perlin, Martin S. *Managing Institutional Planning: Health Facilities and P.L. 93-641.* Germantown, MD: Aspen Systems, 1976.

21. This model is described in Peters, Joseph P.

22. Many readers will agree with Kenneth R. Andrews that "[a board's] detachment from operations equips it to analyze developing strategic decisions with fresh objectivity and breadth of experience. It can be free of the management myopia sometimes produced by operations, in places where keeping things going obscures the directions they are taking." Andrews, p. 171.

23. Andrews, p. 13.

24. Mankin and Glueck, p. 19.

25. For a fuller treatment of the CEO as the "architect of purpose," see Andrews, p. 11 ff.

26. Jackson, Clarence L. Book reviews. *Hospital and Health Services Administration.* 24:103, Fall 1979.

27. Glueck, p. 48.

28. Adapted from a definition by Glueck, p. 8.

29. For more details on SBUs, see Tuller, Edwin, and Kozak, David. Logical thought process key to corporate plan. *Hospitals, J.A.H.A.* 53:82, Sept. 1, 1979. Also see Hofer and Schendel, chapters 5 and 6.

30. Drucker, Peter F. *Management: Tasks—Responsibilities—Practices.* New York City: Harper & Row, Publishers, 1974, p. 77.

31. For more on the idealized-design process inherent in selecting a mission, see Ackoff, Russell L. *Creating the Corporate Future.* New York City: John Wiley & Sons, 1981, chapter 5.

32. Steiner, George A. *Top Management Planning.* New York City: Macmillan Publishing Co., Inc., 1969, p. 324. For a more detailed treatment of the basic thought structure underlying strategic decisions, see Mintzberg, Henry, and others. The structure of "unstructured" decision processes. *Administrative Science Quarterly.* 21:246, June 1976.

33. Tregoe, Benjamin B. Quoted in: Feinberg, Samuel. From where I sit. *Women's Wear Daily.* 141:10, Sept. 5, 1980, p. 10.

34. Rumelt, Richard P. Evaluation of strategy: theory and models. In: Schendel, Dan E., and Hofer, Charles W., editors. *Strategic Management: A New View of Business Policy and Planning.* Boston: Little, Brown and Company, 1979, pp. 198-99.

35. Andrews, p. 25.

36. Henderson, Bruce D. *Henderson on Corporate Strategy.* Cambridge, MA: Abt Books, 1979, p. 40. Also see Ohmae, chapters 7 and 17.

Part 2

Analysis and Diagnosis

Chapter 3

Identifying and Evaluating an Institution's Current Strategy

"What will pass as the current strategy of a company may almost always be deduced from its behavior, but a strategy for a future of changed circumstance may not always be distinguishable from performance in the present. Strategists who do not look beyond present behavior to the future are vulnerable to surprise."

"[An] unstated strategy cannot be tested or contested and is likely therefore to be weak."

—Kenneth R. Andrews, *The Concept of Corporate Strategy*[1]

"The first thing to be said about corporate strategy is that having one is a step forward. Any strategy, once made explicitly, can quickly be evaluated and improved. But if no attempt is ever made to commit it to paper, there is always the danger that the strategy is either incomplete or misunderstood."

—Seymour Tilles, *Business Policy and Strategy: Concepts and Readings*[2]

Every going concern has some notion of where it is headed and how it intends to get there. In short, it has a strategy, however vague or however unarticulated. When an organization recognizes that it must learn to deal more resolutely with changes in its environment to survive, its first step is to examine its current strategy.

Conceptually, this first step can be divided into two related tasks, which in practice are often performed simultaneously: *identifying the present or past strategy and determining if it is the right direction for the future.* For most hospitals neither task is easy, because most hospitals have not thought in strategic terms nor have they found it necessary to devise a formal strategy for directing their affairs.

To identify the current strategy of an ongoing hospital, it may be necessary to analyze a number of documents, policies, programs, and actions that have contributed to shaping the overall management thrust of the institution. In fact, considerable skill and insight may be needed to glean an idea of the institution's strategy from these sources. Nonetheless, with diligent probing, some statements can be uncovered to determine the values or notions that directed the institution's past affairs, even though the resulting strategy may have been just muddling through. Until this task is done, the institution's leaders will not be able to make intelligent decisions in molding a strategy for the future.

What are some readily available materials that a hospital should examine to uncover its current or past strategy? Here is a list—by no means exhaustive—of some obvious sources from which its leaders or staff may be able to piece together what passes for its strategy:

- Mission statement
- Long-range plan
- Annual budgets and accompanying instructions or assumptions used in their preparation
- Annual reports
- Minutes of meetings of the governing board, membership association or corporation, executive committee, joint conference committee, finance committee, long-range planning committee, administrative council, and other groups or task forces concerned with selected aspects of the overall management of the institution
- Policy manuals
- Statements of goals and objectives

But even these may not always disclose an institution's current strategy. In some instances, the strategy can only be assumed from past policies and actions, and even these present difficulties, because there are often considerable differences between what is stated as policy and what is actually carried out in practice. Nonetheless, an institution's aspirations and strategies are usually reflected in what it does and how it does it. When all else fails, the task may require probing the values of top management to identify the overall thrust of the institution.

The Strategy Review

". . . [I]t is obvious that periodically the basic practices of the company must change to deal with changing conditions and competitive capabilities. If this does not happen, then the company becomes the prisoner of its own past successes. It is unable to change course until unsatisfactory results make it obvious to everyone that the strategy should have been changed long before."

"Clearly, strategy must be under constant review; this is a demanding process in which objectivity and thoroughness are extremely difficult to achieve. Obviously, it requires a high degree of executive skill to encourage and manage the process of strategy review. This is more the art of management than the science."

—Bruce D. Henderson, *Henderson on Corporate Strategy*[3]

The following questions may prove useful in identifying an institution's current strategy:[4]

1. Which phrase most accurately describes the hospital's values with respect to the outside world?
    - Don't rock the boat
    - Roll with the punches
    - Plan ahead
    - Dream ahead

2. How does the hospital react to change?
    - Does nothing
    - Rejects or resists change
    - Adapts to change
    - Seeks change
    - Anticipates change
    - Creates a desired future
3. What is the hospital's growth strategy?
    - Exits gracefully
    - Maintains the present position
    - Increases the market share of present services in its traditional service area
    - Grows selectively, specializes in certain services, or caters to defined markets
    - Diversifies by adding new services or products
    - Pursues vertical integration, for example, more primary care, outreach services, or long-term care
    - Converts the hospital or an underutilized unit to another use
    - Closes the facility
4. Strategic thrust: What are the two or three most important driving forces behind the hospital's present direction?
    - Tradition and past successes
    - Outside sanctions and incentives, including reimbursement
    - Medical staff demands and expectations
    - Results (for example, finances or quality of care)
    - Services offered
    - Market forces, including keeping up with the competition
5. What blend of community and service markets best describes the hospital?
    - Selected services to selected populations/markets
    - Selected services to entire service area/market
    - Broad range of services to selected populations/markets
    - Broad range of services to the entire service area/market
    - Specialized or comprehensive services to a regional or a national market, for example, the Mayo Clinic
6. What is the hospital's role in multi-institutional arrangements?
    - Goes it alone
    - Builds on existing teaching or medical school affiliations
    - Is part of a multi-institutional system
    - Links hospital, physicians, and insurance through a prepaid system such as a health maintenance organization
    - Is a systems builder (for example, promotes mergers or acquisitions or provides contract management services)
7. Which three resources are keys to the hospital's success?
    - Medical staff
    - Nursing and allied health personnel
    - Managerial expertise
    - Finances
    - Physical plant
    - Reputation
    - Political clout
    - Community support
8. What is the hospital's target market area?
    - Immediate area surrounding the hospital
    - Entire local community
    - Service area (extends beyond the local community)

- Beyond traditional service area
- Interstate/national
- International

9. Which types of health care services does the hospital provide?
    - Prevention and promotion
    - Primary and ambulatory care
    - Secondary inpatient care
    - Tertiary inpatient care
    - Long-term care
    - Rehabilitation
    - Palliative or hospice
10. What are the bases for determining the quality of care at the hospital?
    - Adequacy of facilities and equipment
    - Quality of nursing care and performance
    - Presence and quality of house staff
    - Quality of medical staff and physician performance
    - Quality of allied health and support staff
    - Organizational coordination and management
    - Overall patient care and patients' reactions
    - Comparable overall care when compared to other local institutions
11. Which phrase best describes the hospital's position with respect to keeping abreast of advances in medical technology?
    - Does not attempt to keep pace with new advances
    - Lags behind other local hospitals
    - Follows the leader
    - Responds quickly to new technology; is usually the leader in its market area
12. What is the hospital's financial strategy?
    - Accepts reimbursement as a limit
    - Maximizes reimbursement
    - Seeks new sources of revenue through diversification
    - Maximizes philanthropic support
13. What is the hospital's approach to managing external affairs?
    - Responds independently (does its "own thing")
    - Responds cooperatively with those who have a stake in the future of the hospital
    - Attempts to influence regulators and outside control groups
    - Forms and joins coalitions
    - Alters the outside world through political action groups, state associations, and other interest groups
14. In what graduate medical education programs does the hospital participate?
    - No programs
    - A limited number of residency programs
    - A broad array of residency/fellowship programs
    - Limited affiliation with a medical school
    - Major affiliation with a medical school
    - Participates in a local medical education consortium
15. What is the hospital's role in nursing education?
    - None
    - Clinical affiliation
    - Diploma nursing school (registered nurse)
    - Licensed practical nurse program
    - Baccalaureate or associate degree program
16. Does the hospital provide formal educational programs or clinical experience for any of the following?

- X-ray technicians
- Laboratory technicians
- Respiratory therapists
- Physical therapists
- Occupational therapists
- Speech therapists
- Recreational therapists
- Dietitians
- Health service administrators
- Other health occupations

17. In what research activities is the hospital involved?
    - No research activities
    - Limited clinical research
    - Broad array of basic and clinical research programs
    - Cooperates with a university or research institute

Every hospital has one or more strategies that determine what it does and where it is headed; otherwise, its management would not be able to answer the above questions, much less be able to guide the affairs of the institution. The basic question is, therefore, not whether a hospital has a strategy, but whether its present strategy is adequate. In short, once an institution's strategy has been identified, however imperfectly, it should be evaluated to determine whether it is right for the institution. Here are some questions that will be useful in making this evaluation:[5]

- Does the strategy fully exploit the challenges and opportunities in the hospital's environment? Specifically, does it enable the institution to meet the health care needs of its local community or market? Does it permit it to satisfy the expectations of its various constituencies (patients, medical staff, employees, and other groups affected by its activities)?
- Is the strategy consistent with the institution's competencies and resource capabilities, both present and future?
- Are the major provisions of the strategy consistent with the mission and general policies of the organization?
- Does the strategy provide a clear sense of direction for the institution's future efforts?
- Does it help the hospital's leaders in deciding on services to be offered and clientele to be served?
- Is it useful in priority decisions for allocating staff, space, and financial resources?
- Is the strategy sufficiently specific to permit measurement of whether or not the hospital is moving in the desired direction?
- Does the strategy have an appropriate time frame?
- Is it sufficiently flexible to deal with rapid or unexpected change? Specifically, does the underlying strategic management process encourage quick adjustments to change?
- Is the strategy appropriate to the personal values and aspirations of top management?
- Does it conform to the institution's shared basic beliefs, its goals, and its underlying "culture"?
- Is it appropriate to the desired level of contributions to society in general and to the institution's local community or market?
- Is the strategy morally and ethically acceptable to society in general and to the local community?
- Is the strategy capable of being communicated to others?
- Is it known at least to the key members of the governing board and top management?
- Is the strategy workable?

The answers to these questions will enable hospital management to decide whether its current strategy is appropriate for a new future. To restate a colorful analogy made by Neil W. Chamberlain, an institution is a complex of organizational interrelationships that can be likened to a ship's crew traveling an unexplored river with many branches and tributaries. Then the strategy is simply the means

Some Advice from a Leader in the Field

A truly effective strategy review will answer these questions to the general satisfaction of the organization:

- Where do we put our priorities in allocating our resources in money and effort?
- What are the major policies that we choose to implement the strategy?
- What are the products and markets in which we choose to compete?
- What critical assumptions are we making about the competition and the environment?
- Exactly what do we expect to do differently or better than our competitors to be successful?''

—Bruce D. Henderson, *Henderson on Corporate Strategy*[6]

the captain uses to keep the ship afloat and in one piece as it moves over time through a constantly changing environment potentially fraught with many perils.[7] If the answers to the above questions are yes, then the institution is ready to move into the uncharted waters of tomorrow, but nonetheless it must always be alert and prepared to adopt a new strategy or to change direction if conditions require it to do so. The chapters that follow describe how the hospital management can do this in a thoughtful manner.

Notes

1. Andrews, Kenneth R. The *Concept of Corporate Strategy.* Homewood, IL: Richard D. Irwin, Inc., 1980, pp. 24, 37.

2. Tilles, Seymour. How to evaluate corporate strategy. In: McCarthy, Daniel J., and others, editors. *Business Policy and Strategy: Concepts and Readings.* Homewood, IL: Richard D. Irwin, Inc., 1979, p. 325.

3. Henderson, Bruce D. *Henderson on Corporate Strategy.* Cambridge, MA: Abt Books, 1979, pp. 37-39.

4. Several of these questions and ideas listed are paraphrased from the following sources: nos. 1 and 2 are based on Ansoff, H. Igor, and others. *From Strategic Planning to Management.* New York City: John Wiley & Sons, 1976; no. 4 is adapted from Tregoe, B., and Zimmerman, J. W. *Top Management Strategy: What It Is and How to Make It Work.* New York City: Simon & Schuster, 1980; no. 10 comes from Georgopoulos, B., and Mann, F. C. *The Community General Hospital.* New York City: Macmillan, 1962; and no. 13 is derived from Galbraith, J. R. *Organizational Design.* Reading, MA: Addison-Wesley Publishing Co., 1977.

5. Adapted from Andrews, pp. 24, 37; and Tilles, p. 325.

6. Henderson, p. 39.

7. Chamberlain, Neil W. *Enterprise and Environment: The Firm in Time and Place.* New York City: McGraw-Hill, Inc., 1968, pp. 5-6.

Chapter 4

Assessing and Monitoring the External Environment

"Every organization functions in a dual setting: the microenvironment, made up of customers, markets, related industries, and competitors, and a macroenvironment, a four-dimension overlay of societal, government, economic, and technological forces that affect the organization's operations."

—William E. Rothschild, *Putting It All Together: A Guide to Strategic Thinking*[1]

"Often, in our business, we think of environment as something 'out there' that causes problems for us, often dramatically, and usually unpredictably. Perhaps we could better relate to environmental change if we altered our views of the relationships involved. For, in reality, environment is not something 'out there' constraining us. Environment is something we are a part of, and environmental constraints are the interacting relationships that we must manage."

—William F. Christopher, *Management for the 1980s*[2]

"The most important single influence on organizational policy and strategy is the environment outside and inside the organization. The more complex, turbulent, and changing is the environment, the greater is its impact on human attitudes, organizational structures, and processes. Since today's environment has rarely been exceeded in complexity, turbulence, rapidity of change, and significance of change, all organizations, large and small, for their survival must pay more attention than ever before to their environments when formulating and implementing policies and strategies."

—George A. Steiner and John B. Miner, *Management Policy and Strategy*[3]

If an institution is to survive and prosper in the future, two questions must be asked repeatedly by hospital management: What is going on in the world? How will it affect us? Hospital CEOs and trustees are not accustomed to asking these questions, at least not in the sense of concentrating their attention on external forces and developments. By inclination and training, they are more concerned with internal management, a task certainly deserving constant attention and best efforts. They tend to think in terms of holding things together, keeping things going, and fixing things.[4] Therefore, it is understandable that few of them have the time or the energy to worry about developments outside of the organization, particularly when they recognize that often very little can be done to control or influence these external forces. Yet there are many things happening in the outside world that should concern hospital management.

Every organization exists in a dual environment of space and time that influences everything it does or aspires to do. This environment is the pattern of all the external conditions and factors that affect its life, its structure, its basic policies, and its development.[5] It includes various economic, technological, political, legal, societal, psychological, demographic, and market forces that can limit an organization's activities, provide it with new opportunities, or threaten its well being. In fact, "It may be clearer and more accurate to recognize environments in the plural sense, for the environment of an institution is composed of numerous elements and forces which act and react to the benefit or detriment of the organization."[6]

To cope with these pressing external influences, management must learn to view its efforts from an ecological perspective, *from the outside in.* Perceptive managers realize that only when the external environment is understood and managed successfully can an organization grow or possibly even survive. Getting the job done efficiently is no longer enough; managers must also think in terms of managing change.

To think strategically, management must learn how to be alert to changes in the outside environment by conducting what is variously termed an *environmental assessment, an environmental analysis, an environmental scanning,* or an *external analysis.* Regardless of the term used to describe this activity, it is simply the means by which management identifies, appraises, monitors, and forecasts various events and trends that may have an impact on an organization's choice of strategy and on how it carries out the strategy. Its purpose is to detect early signs of potential change, to understand these changes, and to make the organization aware of the implication of these changes on its future direction. In short, it provides an outside-in perspective that enables the organization to pinpoint possible areas of future opportunity and trouble.

Assessments Must Lead to Operating Implications

"The real value to an organization of any systematic assessment of 'environmental' factors lies in the *operating implications* which the organization draws for itself from that assessment. An organization must ask and answer the question, 'What *specifically* does this mean to us in terms of our operations?' Failure to extend an 'environmental assessment' to its operating implications for an organization severely limits the usefulness of the assessment process."

—*Strategic Challenges for the Eighties: An Environmental Assessment of the Health Care Industry in the Upper Midwest*[7]

Environmental Assessment

At the outset, a decision should be made about when and how often management will conduct external assessments. Should they be made on an ad hoc basis, for example, when clear opportunities or threats present themselves, or should they be conducted on a more regular basis? The answer depends in large measure on the nature of the environment. In tranquil times when change is slow and its impact on an organization is easily managed, being alert to outside changes may not be important. In today's turbulent times, however, the need to monitor the outside environment is greater than ever before and promises to grow. If hospitals are to survive and flourish, their leaders must learn to integrate ongoing environmental scanning efforts into the management process as an essential first step in handling external change.

The ad hoc external analyses conducted by the 12 best thinkers or other top-level participants at special two-day retreats should not be played down. These retreats have proven effective in getting a strategic management activity underway. However, it should be recognized that these retreats are not one-shot efforts. Retreats are simply forerunners of the continuous scanning activities that must subsequently be conducted as an essential ingredient of good hospital management.

Some suggestions for developing an environmental scanning, assessment, and monitoring system follow. They will enable a hospital to develop an aggressive and entrepreneurial strategic management program.

- Organize a systematic procedure for early identification of outside opportunities and threats.
- Make arrangements for managing these tasks on a continuing basis.
- Assign staff to carry out these tasks and hold management responsible for assessing the importance and implications of the findings.
- Devise a system for ensuring a quick, upward flow of information on external developments and changes to allow top management to respond rapidly to problems that may arise from any source: economic, political, social, or technological.
- Keep these arrangements compatible with the existing organizational structure and with internal management information systems.

Five separate but interrelated tasks are involved in carrying out an environmental assessment:

- Scanning the environment for early signs of emerging changes and trends that may have an impact on the institution
- Understanding best as one can the various forces that create these changes
- Monitoring and tracking change on a continuing basis
- Forecasting what will happen as a result of change
- Developing arrangements to ensure that the environmental assessment gets to the right persons in time for them to take appropriate action

Write It Down!

"The first step in the strategic planning process is a written assessment of the operating environment of the industry of which the organization is a part. . . . For instance, the American Hospital Association had to determine what major external factors would influence the hospital industry in the future, and what opportunities and problems these factors are likely to present to the AHA. By preparing a written environmental assessment, an organization is able to ensure that these questions will be answered more comprehensively than might otherwise be the case given the press of day-to-day activities. Because the external environment is subject to change, these questions must be answered on a regular basis. A written environmental assessment provides the basis for regular updates. Finally, a written environmental assessment is a valuable communications device, because it provides an opportunity for all elements of the organization to start from a common base of information and allows disagreements with respect to external factors and their impact on the organization to be addressed prior to the development of plan and budgets."

—Edwin Tuller and David Kozak,
Hospitals, J.A.H.A.[8]

Several "tricks of the trade" are helpful in carrying out these various tasks and have proven their worth in a variety of hospital and nonhospital situations:

Learn to think in terms of multilevel analysis: worldwide, national, industrywide, regional, state, and local. The energy crisis is a good example of *worldwide* social-political-economic-technological trends that have a universal impact. Many overriding *national* economic, social, and other factors affect not only health care services in general, but also individual hospitals, their patients, and their communities. Inflation, high interest rates, and the growing disarray of political liberalism are some recent examples. These, in turn, may influence the *hospital industry* as a whole, although the industry itself may also be changing as the result of new ideas and developments from within. The growth of multihospital systems, the application of marketing principles, the growing sensitivity to the special needs of the dying and the terminally ill, and the emphasis on health promotion and disease prevention are examples. In addition, geopolitical perspectives at the *regional or multistate* level often reflect different attitudes or political leanings, which can shape what a health care organization does and how it does it. The distribution of medical groups and physicians participating in groups, for example, varies considerably by region: the ratio of group practitioners to population in the West is almost twice that of the Northeast.[9] Health care resources and their sponsorship also vary noticeably by and within regions. Of course, it is at *state and community levels* where the greatest variations in values, emphases, and resource capabilities are evident. It is at the local level that health care is sought, delivered, received, and ultimately paid for. For these reasons, hospitals and other health care providers focus most of their planning and marketing assessments on their local communities.

Make a distinction between controllable and uncontrollable trends and events. The former call for preventive measures; the latter require contingency thinking. Much time can be wasted on uncontrollable situations.

Do not move in too many directions; focus on the most important trends or events. A wise approach is to take a broad sweep of what is going on externally and then to focus on several key happenings and developments that promise to have the greatest impact on the institution and on various persons who can influence what the institution does or does not do.

Be alert to events that can trigger other events that may affect the institution. For example, if a government study were to report that coffee is bad for the pancreas, the coffee industry would have good cause to worry. Federal budget cuts or legislation requiring more restrictive Medicaid entitlement benefits could alter payments for hospital services, and, in turn, these could precipitate financial problems for hospitals. Similar forces, such as the changing position of women in society, can affect career choices and possibly result in a decline in the number of women pursuing health careers. Although individual institutions can do very little to influence these events or forces, they can develop strategies to minimize their impact.

Search for changes in underlying conditions. Thinking in terms of the multidimensional overlay of trends and events described above and recognizing the interdependence of factors can be helpful. Another approach is to determine the rules of the game that govern the hospital industry. Are these changing? How will the new rules affect the industry as a whole? How will they affect individual institutions and various stakeholders? For example, is the hospital industry moving away from cooperation, which emphasizes the public good, to competition, which promotes institutional interests? What *underlying forces* are driving this change? How would this shift affect individual institutions and local communities? Will new strategies be requried? Thinking in terms of broad underlying change is not easy. It requires a habit of disciplined thinking that is either learned through education or developed through experience—a habit of not accepting the obvious as a necessary cause, of carefully examining and questioning the many facets of change, of exercising a healthy skepticism, and of regarding most analyses as tentative.

Some Advice on Using Informal Networks

"Effective change managers actively develop informal networks to get objective information—from other staff and line executives, workers, customers, board members, suppliers, politicians, technologists, educators, outside professionals, government groups, and so on—to sense possible needs for change. They purposely use these networks to short-circuit all the careful screens their organizations build up to 'tell the top only what it wants to hear'. . . . Since people sift signals about threats and opportunities through perceptual screens defined by their own values, careful executives make sure their sensing networks include people who look at the world very differently than do those in the enterprise's dominating culture. Effective executives consciously seek options and threat signals beyond the *status quo*. 'If I'm not two or three years ahead of my organization, I'm not doing my job' was a common comment of such executives in the sample."

—James Brian Quinn, *Sloan Management Review*[12]

Look for early signals. Some events can develop so rapidly or are so unexpected that they arrive unannounced and surprise institutions. H. Igor Ansoff warns that managers must learn to cope with "strategic surprises" by increasing their reliance on "weak signals."[10] James Brian Quinn emphasizes this advice by observing that "early signals may come from anywhere and may be difficult to distinguish from the background 'noise' of ordinary communications. Crises, of course, announce themselves with strident urgency in operations control systems. But, if organizations wait until signals reach amplitudes high enough to be sensed by formal measurement systems, smooth, efficient transitions may be impossible."[11]

Thinking in terms of future events having serious ramifications is a habit not easily acquired. Persons tend to filter signals about trends and events through perceptions that reflect their backgrounds, training, and values. Their perspective of what is ahead is often so short-ranged that they become aware of what's happening only when it personally affects them or the organization. Executives in particular must learn how to step outside these limitations and become sensitive to possibilities that are still in the incubation stage.[13] Those who are alert to early signals often are able to take anticipatory action long before their competitors, thereby capitalizing on opportunities for new markets, new products, and new venture operations.

Discover the issues that should be addressed. Many issues, such as overbedding, consolidation, regulation, and diversification, are being debated. They will help define and determine the basic nature and direction of a hospital. There are also human issues, such as care of the indigent or abortion, that trouble persons who have a stake in the hospital activities. Identifying these can be difficult, and they are often obtained only through careful interviewing of a broad cross-section of affected parties.[14]

Learn how to treat future uncertainty. Much of what will take place in the future is "iffy" and the would-be strategist must be prepared to confront the unknown or the uncertain. Many ways of handling an uncertain future exist; some alternatives are to forget it, forecast a range of possibilities, think in terms of contingency planning, devise some alternative futures, conduct a what-if analysis, or, if all else fails, hang loose.

Do not be afraid to face up to bad tidings. Falling prey to the Persian Messenger syndrome of punishing the bearer of bad news is easy. However, according to William S. Woodside, "You should lean over backwards to reward the guy who is first with the bad news."[15] Not only can the bad news save an organization's life by averting or lessening the impact of outside threats, it can also give the organization a timely advantage over its competitors who may be equally vulnerable to the same threats. However, the threat must be recognized before any preventive action can be taken.

Where does hospital management obtain information about what is happening in the outside world? How does it analyze and apply this information? At the outset, information is valuable in handling external influences, be they threats, opportunities, or challenges. However, information is not always available or good and, therefore, cannot be an absolute prerequisite to making sound strategic decisions; if this were so, few such decisions would ever be made. The trick is to use the knowledge at hand, realize its limitations, and increase that knowledge by reading, attending meetings, and above all, talking to knowledgeable persons.[16]

Little excuse exists for any hospital executive to be uninformed about major developments in the health care field. Numerous journals, futures-oriented consumer studies and policy analyses, survey services, and seminars and workshops are geared toward developments in the hospital and related health care fields. However, selecting programs best suited to a specific situation can be a problem. Talking to colleagues about the merits of a specific conference or about the competence of the faculty can be helpful in making such choices.

Acquiring, Applying, and Communicating the Findings

"For the organization wishing to examine its environment, substantial volumes of data are at hand. Acquiring the information, however, is far less difficult and interesting than is examining it and making it relevant to corporate decision making. In particular, the problem is getting the attention of the corporate decision-makers.

"The person charged with the responsibility for environmental analysis has two principal tasks. First, he must be aware of, and have access to, techniques and organizations making the studies and measurements. . . . But of equal importance is his understanding of the decision-making process in his own organization, and his awareness of the decisons being considered and made within that organization. It is only through that understanding and awareness that the analyst will be able to select from the flood of reports, notes, publications, and other input what particular data are useful for which organizational decisions."

—Rene D. Zentner, *The Journal of Business Strategy*[17]

Techniques

Several approaches and techniques, if used judiciously, will enable management to identify and monitor the various environmental forces that influence an institution's future. This identification and monitoring process is as good a way as any to get a strategic thinking process underway; it is certainly an essential early step in developing an organization's strategy and in devising specific plans to carry out the strategy. Unfortunately, the state of the art is not yet well developed, and a single best method to which an organization can turn does not exist.[18] Each hospital should select the tools most appropriate to its own situation.

What is important is that, in some systematic manner, management scrutinizes those outside forces, issues, and developments that the techniques are designed to identify. Therefore any or all of the following tools should be tailored to a hospital's own needs and should be augmented with new methods (see figure 2, Selected Techniques That Link an Organization with Environmental Change).

Trend evaluation and monitoring. Many hospitals rely on general and trade publications to keep abreast of developments that may affect their operations. Many do this in a casual and unstructured manner. CEOs, middle management, and department heads screen a few items that come to their attention and either make use of the information at once or retain it to be used later, if needed. The weaknesses of this approach are obvious: it neither ensures that important items will be read and analyzed nor does it guarantee that the information will be used to meet needs and problems as they arise.

Of course, these uncertainties can be reduced by structuring the flow of information throughout the organization and by devising ways for bringing the information to management's attention on a regular basis. This is usually done by assigning the task to an in-house planner, a librarian, or some other staff member who carries out the role of resident futurist. Keeping a file of relevant clippings, articles, and notes titled "Happenings That May Affect Us" can be helpful in focusing attention on external change. These can be duplicated and circulated to other members of the management team to whom it would be useful.

Two examples of how organizations identify and monitor potential issues for the future are well known by their acronyms: TAP, the Trend Analysis Program, and TEAM, Trend Evaluation and Monitoring. A major advantage of both approaches is that they draw on individual firms to identify trends and issues, thereby overcoming in part the tunnel vision, lethargy, or resistance that some companies display in handling external change.[19]

Environmental trend analysis. This technique for identifying and assessing environmental change is usually performed as part of a two-day retreat or other special occasion at which key representatives of a hospital's governing board, medical staff, and administration or its 12 best thinkers assemble to discuss future strategies. The technique is simple. The participants are instructed to select the three or four most critical trends and implications within various environmental categories (see figure 3, Environmental Trend Analysis). If the group is large, it can be divided into subgroups, with each working group assigned a particular environmental category, for example, political or technological developments. The results are then presented to the entire group for consideration.

Stakeholder analysis. Many persons who are not informed about the details of hospital operation tend to limit a hospital's constituency to its patients, employees, and medical staff. But many outside groups—new stakeholders—have an interest or say in the institution's affairs and may be affected by what the institution does—or fails to do. Good management strategy recognizes the special significance of the concept of stakeholders. It is particularly relevant in turbulent times when management must learn to handle an institution's broadening, vocal, and at times, hostile constituencies and their changing roles, needs, expectations, and demands.

The first step is to identify those groups, either internal or external to the institution, whose *collective action* can directly affect the institution, but whose behavior is not under the institution's direct control. Management should also keep in mind that stakeholders not only provide inputs, they also expect and sometimes control outputs.

The second step involves analyzing each stakeholder group in terms of what it wants now or may want in the future, how the institution interacts with the group, and what the various trends and expected changes are that sustain and shape the relationship between the organization and the particular group (see figure 4, Stakeholder Analysis). This information forms the basis for converting stakeholder expectations into institutional strategies and objectives.[20]

Analysis of competition. An important element of a hospital's external environment is its local competition—other hospitals and health care providers that serve the same community or medical market. Therefore identification and assessment of that competition are essential early in the development of an institution's strategic management effort (see figure 5, How to Do a Simple Competitive Analysis).

The following basic questions are helpful in conducting an analysis:[22]

- Who are the hospital's competition and who will they be in the future? Are any new entrants expected?
- What are the hospital's key competitor's strategies, missions, and plans?
- What unique strengths and resources do the hospital's competitors possess? Are these likely to change in the future?
- Do they have any weaknesses that make them especially vulnerable?
- How important is a specific service area, clientele, or market to these competitors and are they committed enough to continue to invest more resources into serving this market?
- What activities or changes are the hospital's competitors involved in or planning, for example, changes in mission and direction, programs, management, or patient mix; addition or curtailment of services; acquisition of specialized equipment and high technology; new construction or relocation; satellite operations; zealous recruitment of nurses or medical staff; new or expanded educational programs; cut-throat competition, and mergers or acquisitions?
- What are the implications of any or all of the above for the hospital? On the local hospital industry? On the local medical market? On the local job market? On meeting the community's health service needs?

The key to this analysis is to think in terms of the past, present, and future challenges and threats presented by the most important direct competitors. Part of good management rests in its ability to question why some institutions always seem to be out front, whereas others seem content to be followers.[23] Dynamic strategic management allows an institution to prepare strategies for placing itself in a new competitive position. Knowing the competition is a necessary first step in accomplishing this.

Michael E. Porter has devised a helpful schema that recognizes that competitive forces go well beyond the usual combatants in a particular industry or market. In his view, customers, suppliers, potential entrants, and substitute products are all competitors that may be more or less prominent or active depending on the industry. His schema diagrams five basic forces: *the threat of new entrants, the bargaining power of customers, the bargaining power of suppliers, the threat of substitute (or new) products or services, and the jockeying for position among current competitors within the industry or local market.*[24] (See figure 6, Forces Governing Competition in an Industry.) Porter's schema is a useful tool in stimulating analysis and discussion at strategic retreats and at other group sessions where participants identify competitive and related environmental forces in an industry or local health care market that promise to have an impact on the work of their institution. A review of the five basic forces discloses the value of Porter's approach to an analysis of competition.

New entrants to a market bring new capacities that can disturb existing arrangements. For example, the intention to erect the 777-bed City of Faith Hospital in the purportedly overbedded market of Tulsa, OK, provoked consternation and subsequent legal action among existing local hospitals. Areawide health planning agencies have also been preoccupied with the threat of new entrants. Indeed, the health planning movement and much of the legislation that has supported it have been based on the recognition that in many instances new entrants would unnecessarily duplicate existing services, compete for scarce personnel and financial resources, and contribute to the rising costs of health care. And yet, although the barriers to entry are high in the hospital field and newcomers must be capable of mobilizing considerable financial resources and attracting many qualified professionals, new hospital and related health ventures crop up whenever state certificate-of-need regulators allow them. Monitoring these developments is an important element in an environmental assessment.

Selected Techniques That Link an Organization with Environmental Change

Technique/ Elements	Trend Evaluation and Monitoring (TEAM)	Environmental Trend Analysis	Stakeholder Analysis	Analysis of Competition
Starting point	Signals of change in publications and reports	Participants' identification of selected critical trends and implications	Stakeholders who affect or will be affected by organization's actions	Determination of present and future competition
What is it?	A participative strategic scanning process	A participative work session usually held during a retreat or special workshop	Analysis of constituencies with whom organization must deal	Identification and assessment of competitors and how they are likely to affect organization
Key ideas, steps	Gather information by monitoring publications Utilize information (staff, strategic planning committee, top management)	Conduct free-wheeling discussion of three or four most critical trends identified by participants Analyze implications of trends; identify changes that might affect the future direction of organization	Identify stakeholders' expectations and demands and their change over time Do management values reflect these expectations?	Identify direct competitors, possible new entrants Specify their role, plans, and strategies; their strengths and weaknesses List implications

Technique/ Elements	Competitive Position Analysis	Vulnerability Analysis	Environmental Threat and Opportunity Profile (ETOP)	Issues Alert Matrix
Starting point	Determination of where we stand in relation to the competition	Compilation of underpinnings and basic beliefs	Need to identify and assess important external factors	Exploration of the expected probability and impact of various changes
What is it?	A systematic evaluation to determine market strength	Assessment of threats to underpinnings of the organization	A systematic diagnostic and weighing of environmental threats and opportunities	Assessment of probability and impact of outside changes
Key ideas, steps	Consider following factors: market share and position, pricing policy, degree of integration, financial position, product mix, technological capability, quality of services, marketing capabilities	Identify underpinnings Identify threats Assess threats Display results	Participants or staff weigh various factors and measure potential impact on organization Factors weighed from +5 (strongly positive) to 0 (neutral) to −5 (strongly negative) Very high impact (+50) to neutral/no impact (0) to serious threat (−50)	Plot probability (high, medium, low) and impact (high, medium, low) of various expected changes

Figure 2. Comparing aspects of these techniques will help a hospital choose a method tailored to its specific needs.

Environmental Trend Analysis

Instructions

List the environmental factors and changes that should be considered in establishing the future direction of the hospital. Using this information, available background information, and your own experience and knowledge, select the three or four most critical trends and implications for the environmental categories assigned to your group.

For each category:

1. Review, amend, and make additions to the trends.
2. Draw out implications of the trends, looking particularly for changes that might make an impact on the future direction of the hospital, offering opportunities or threats.
3. Select three or four threats and opportunities that in your judgment are *critical* to the future of the hospital.

Worksheet

Category:____________________

Trends	Implications	Critical Threats and Opportunities

Figure 3. This worksheet facilitates conducting an environmental trend analysis during a retreat or other special meeting.

Stakeholder Analysis

Stakeholder____________________

Item	Description	Analysis
Scale and importance	Estimated numbers of the group Judgment as to relative importance	
Stakeholder concerns	How dependent are they on us? What does the group contribute? How do they hope to benefit? Why do they behave as they do?	
Concerns of the organization	To what extent are we dependent on them? What do we expect from the group?	
Social, political, technological, and economic context	What external trends and changes underlie, shape, and have an impact on the interaction between the organization and the stakeholder?	
Issues	Areas of issue, controversy, unmet expectations, changing directions, impact of the organization's strategy and/or actions	

Figure 4. The information to be added to this worksheet forms the basis for converting stakeholder expectations into institutional strategies.[21]

How to Do a Simple Competitive Analysis

1. Select three or four direct competitors. Develop the following information:
   - Hospital strategy (growth, service, markets, and positioning)
   - Multi-institutional arrangements
   - New initiatives
   - Vulnerabilities
   - Resources (plant, medical staff, trustees, and management)
   - Financial condition
   - Services
   - Patients
2. List sources for competitive information:

Figure 5. Following the instructions in this form will provide information needed to conduct a competitive analysis.

Forces Governing Competition in an Industry

Michael E. Porter states that the nature and degree of competition in an industry hinge on five forces: the threat of new entrants, the bargaining power of customers, the bargaining power of suppliers, and the jockeying among current contestants.

1. ______________________________

____

____

____

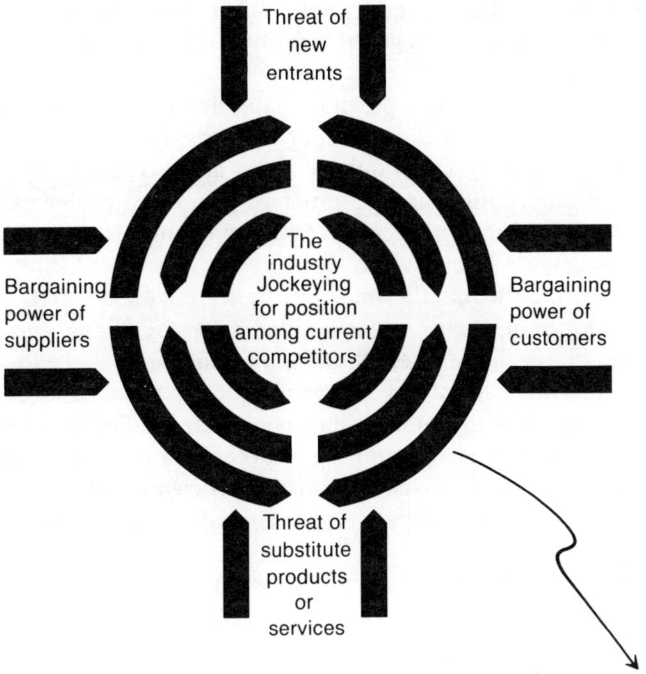

2. _______________

____

____

____

____

____

3. _______________

____

____

____

____

____

4. ______________________________

____

____

____

5. ______________________

____

____

____

Figure 6. This figure illustrates how five competitive forces shape a hospital's strategy.

Customers and *suppliers* can exert considerable bargaining power by influencing prices and the quality and scope of available services. Patients and other purchasers of health care services can, at times, force institutions to supply certain desired services and even specify how and where these will be offered. Physicians, in particular, exercise a powerful influence on almost everything a hospital does, both as customers, who have the sole power to admit patients and to order various diagnostic and treatment services, and as suppliers, who actually provide these services.

Many other readily familiar groups, such as Blue Cross and other prepaid health insurers and government third-party payers, collectively account for perhaps as much as 90 percent or more of a hospital's operating revenue. These large-scale purchasers usually require that participating institutions adhere to specified quality, procedural, and accounting standards. These, in turn, can affect the supplying institution's services and costs. These large-scale purchasers of hospital services as yet are not prone to shop for favorable prices or to play one supplier against another as often happens in other business situations. However, this may change in a more competitive environment.

More important than the threat of new entrants or the other competitive forces already mentioned is the *threat of substitute or new products and services.* Actually, much of the competition that takes place among hospitals assumes this form. Some institutions seem always to be leaders. They are usually the first in their communities to acquire new technology, offer new programs, or provide substitute services. Whether they do so to better serve their markets, to satisfy the expectations of their medical staffs, or simply to seek a competitive edge may not be clear. Nonetheless, their actions can threaten other health service institutions, often triggering responses by neighboring facilities to adopt similar strategies.

In addition, hospitals are already under pressure to develop less costly alternatives to hospitalization and many of them have inaugurated ambulatory surgery, home health care, long-term institutional care, and wellness programs.[25] Other outside forces are also pressuring health care facilities to change their basic roles.[26] This cautious competition may pose many problems and difficulties to laggard institutions that are unwilling or unprepared to adopt counter strategies to retain their share of the local health care market.

Hospitals *jockey for position* within their markets by employing a variety of tactics. Some compete vigorously for physicians and other scarce personnel by offering various salary and benefit incentives, loan guarantees, tuition assistance, subsidized housing, and other inducements. Indeed, some hospitals seem prepared to take almost any competitive action short of an advertising "slugfest."

Interhospital rivalries exist in many multihospital communities. For the most part, these are more benign than hostile and do not impede or discourage local cooperative arrangements. Because hospitals are part of a mature industry, time has helped eliminate inefficient, irrelevant, or obsolete institutions that are unable to adapt to changing conditions. In occasional instances, competition may have simply dealt the final blow.

With the present trend toward fewer but larger facilities and the continuing growth of large investor-owned chains, the lessening of interhospital rivalries or of additional closures and acquisitions of inefficient institutions is unlikely. Indeed, jockeying for position may become more aggressive as hospitals compete for patients, physicians, and resources in a more permissive competitive environment. Therefore, an analysis of competition using Porter's schema or some other appropriate tool will continue to be a key element in carrying out a hospital environmental assessment.

Competitive position analysis. This analysis is a variation of the previous technique. As its proponents Darryl J. Ellis and Peter P. Pekar Jr. indicate, "It is useful to think of the competitive position of a distinct business area as being one of the following: dominant, strong, advantageous, vulnerable, or insignificant. Knowing where one stands with respect to the competition is essential for determining the strategic options available."[27] Considerable information about each competitor's activities, programs, resources, staffing, finances, and market share is required to complete this analysis (see figure 7, Competitive Position Analysis Worksheet).

Methods for defining a hospital's geographic service area, its market, vary in terms of sophistication and complexity. Most hospitals regularly compile information on where their patients come from by conducting a patient residence study.[28] This is, of course, useful in specifying the institution's service area, but it tells little or nothing about its share of that market. Because no one hospital has total information about where the inhabitants of its service area receive hospital care, a coordinated and cooperative effort of all hospitals serving that area is needed. Admissions or discharges for all hospitals from a given area, city, or county are tabulated and distributed by hospitals, making it possible to determine each hospital's importance in serving the area, an essential piece of information for any market comparison.

An actual example based on a recent study by one of the co-authors follows. A sampling of 632 admissions disclosed that 60.4 percent of the hospital's patients reside in its immediate community. However, cooperative Professional Activity Study data showed that the hospital accounted for only 1,239, or 20.6 percent, of the 6,028 persons from its local area who were hospitalized during the past year in hospitals throughout its county. Obviously, this hospital is not the major hospital resource for its community, even though it is the only hospital located in that particular community. Some new strategies are required if the institution hopes to strengthen its market position.[29]

Much information is also available from state and metropolitan hospital associations, health planning bodies, state licensing agencies, third-party payers, and annual reports and other documents issued by local hospitals. It can also be obtained by talking to colleagues and particularly to physicians who have local joint hospital appointments. In general, this information is usually shared among institutions, often on a regular basis and sometimes only on request. In a more competitive environment, this willingness to share information and statistical data could lessen.

Vulnerability analysis. Every organization has certain qualities, resources, and values on which it bases its programs and which enable it to carry out its business. The developer of vulnerability analysis, SRI International, terms it the *underpinnings* of the operation. As with many other basic aspects of life, these are often taken for granted. Only when the organization is threatened by outside change or when the system breaks down internally are these basic dependencies made explicit and analyzed.

Some of the more obvious factors that form the underpinnings of a hospital are the needs and expectations of patients, resources and assets, the physician base, the caliber of its employees, technologies, quality of services, local acceptance (goodwill), community values, institutional identity and reputation, integrity of service, stability of costs with respect to the market, and institutional philosophy and values (its basic beliefs). A good management strategy is to identify and analyze potential threats and challenges to these underpinnings (see figure 8, Vulnerability Analysis: A Threat Assessment).[30] Indeed, once management learns to think in outside-in terms, it will often find itself conducting such an analysis. This analysis certainly should be done whenever outside forces threaten the institution or when management inaugurates a strategic management effort.

Environmental threat and opportunity profile (ETOP). How significant are the various outside forces that promise to influence an organization's future? Several of the preceding tools are designed to identify these forces and to assist management in assessing their impact. However, to do this effectively, William F. Glueck suggests a more systematic approach: ETOP is a technique for weighing various environmental factors that have an impact either as threats or opportunities on an organization and its activities.[31]

Participants or staff rate various factors that have been identified by some other tool, such as trend evaluation and monitoring or environmental trend analysis, by applying the following scales:

> From +5 (strongly positive) to 0 (neutral) to -5 (strongly negative)
> to weigh the *importance* of each factor
>
> From +50 (very high opportunity) to 0 (neutral or no impact) to -50 (serious threat)
> to determine *impact* of each factor

This technique can be refined and made as detailed and as specific as desired. It can also be incorporated into a Delphi analysis (see chapter 5).

Issues alert matrix. This matrix is easy to use for portraying and assessing the probability and impact of various environmental issues and changes on an organization (see figure 9, Issues Alert Matrix). A development such as a shortage of registered nurses, state rate review, or less regulation or market entry (certificate of need) is plotted in terms of its probability of future occurrence and its impact on

Competitive Position Analysis Worksheet

Description	Your Area	Major Competitors (Name)	Potential Competitors
Percent of market share: volume (percent of admissions, patient days, ER visits, etc.) dollar basis (actual/estimated share of total hospital expenditures)			
Change in market share in recent years (specify)			
Estimated future market share in next 3 years			
Utilization (average daily census, occupancy percentage, average length of stay)			
Scope of services (broad or narrow)			
Strong services			
Degree of market concentration			
Character of medical staff			
Reputation in community (outstanding, good, average, or poor)			

Figure 7. This worksheet is a useful tool in compiling the information required to perform a competitive position analysis.

Figure 7 (continued)

Financial position (favorable or unfavorable)
Financial reserves (specify)
Financial performance (surplus or deficit)
Cost per patient day (amount)
Outside contributions (amount)
Debt service (amount)
Technological innovation and capability (strong, average, or weak)
Employee morale (good, average, or poor)
Employee turnover (high, average, or low)
Patient satisfaction (good, average, or poor)
Other factors (specify)
OVERALL RATING*

*Note: In preparing overall rating, rate your institution and each competitor as follows:

- *Dominant.* Controls behavior of other competitors; has a wide choice of strategic options.
- *Strong.* Can take independent action without jeopardizing its position or resources, and able to maintain it regardless of competitor's actions.
- *Advantageous.* Has exploitable strengths greater than average opportunity to improve market position.
- *Vulnerable.* Sufficiently satisfactory performance to continue in operation, but has a less than average opportunity to improve position.
- *Insignificant.* Unsatisfactory performance, but opportunity exists for improvement; usually must change if it is to survive.

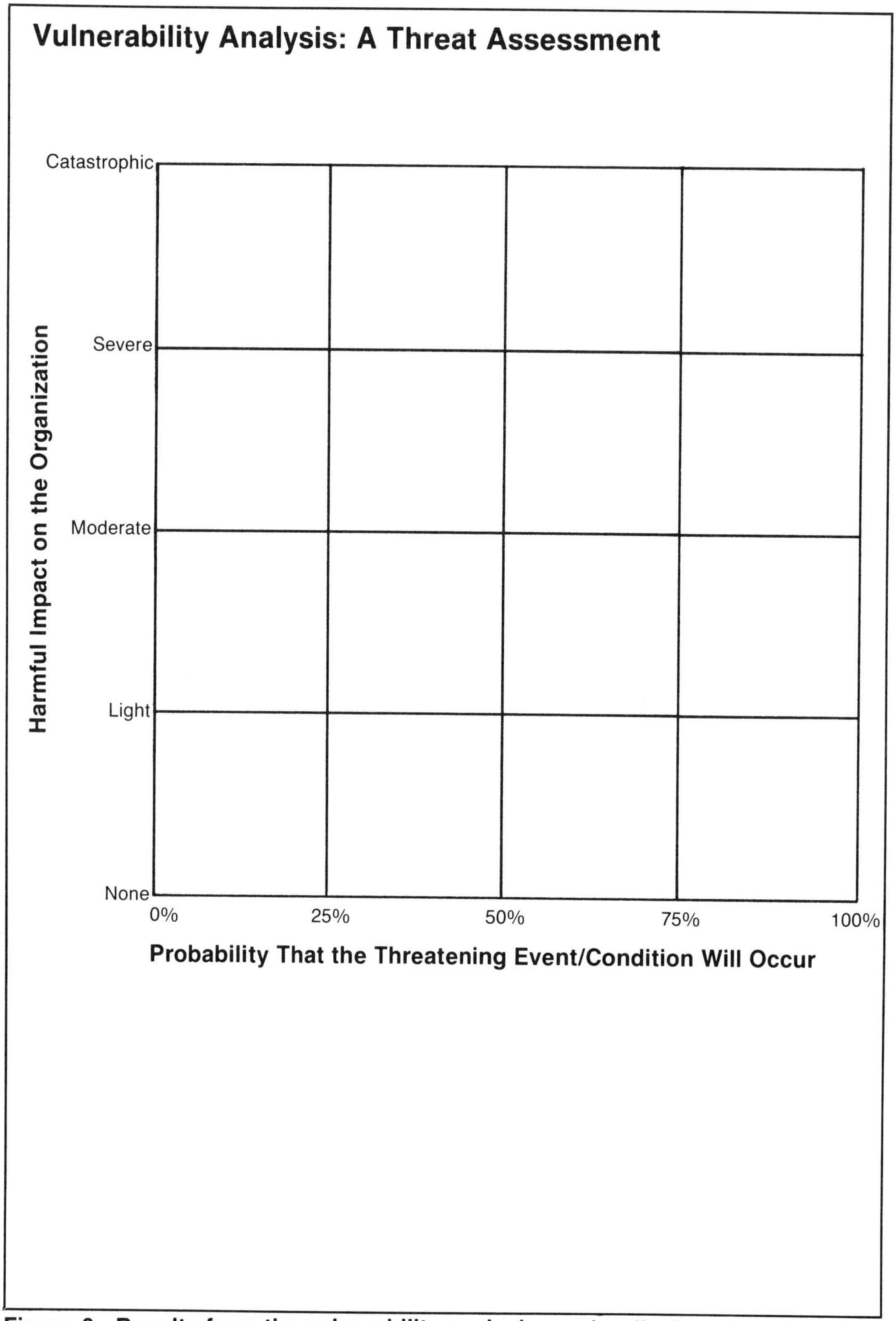

Figure 8. **Results from the vulnerability analysis can be displayed to show the likelihood of the event occurring and how strong the impact will be on the hospital.**

Issues Alert Matrix

The environmental analysis results can be portrayed in an issues alert matrix.[33]

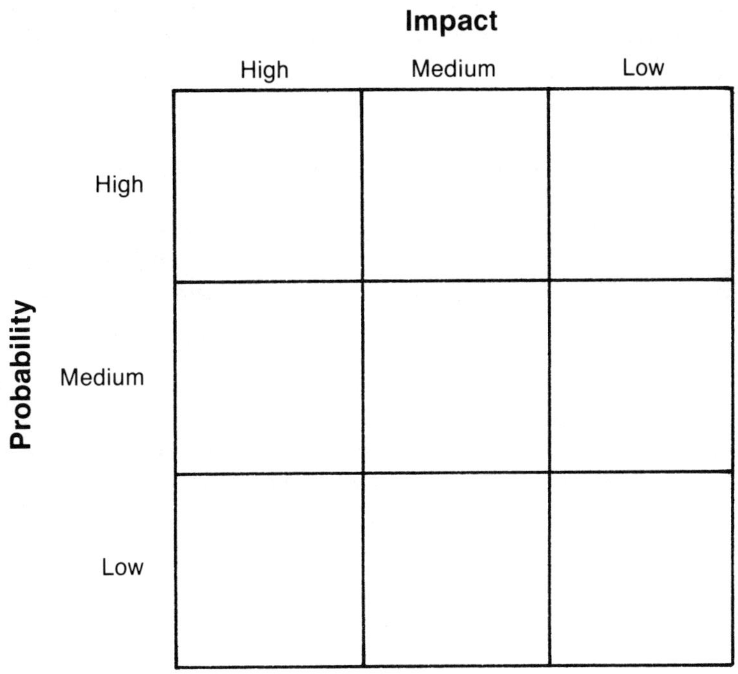

To provide a sense of timing, a matrix can be drawn for several points in time.

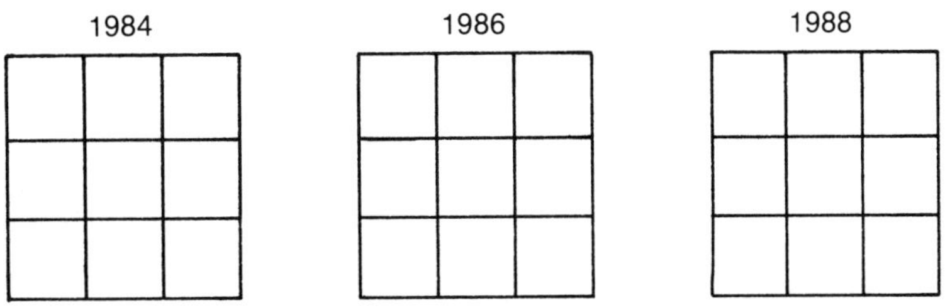

Figure 9. The issues alert matrix portrays and assesses the probability and impact of environmental changes on an organization.

the institution. This technique enables management to focus its attention on those outside developments that are most likely to take place and that promise to have a large impact. To provide a sense of timing, matrixes can be drawn at several points in time. This tool is extremely useful at a retreat or other special occasion during which the participants make a conscious effort to weigh the impact of present and future developments.

Each of the techniques discussed in this chapter helps to focus management's attention on some aspect of the environment. Some provide early warning signals with sufficient lead time for opportunistic action; others focus on changes about which management can do little, except figure out how to avert or minimize potential negative impacts.

As management becomes more sensitive to outside influences, it will also discover that the outside world is complex. Undesired repercussions can occur when intervening with outside change, and, therefore, management should not be frustrated if events do not always work out as planned or if past strategies that were well prepared fail. Of course, this should not discourage management from trying to better position the organization in its environment or develop strategies in the face of uncertainty. It simply means that management must become more alert and more adept in preparing for and handling the uncertain and the unexpected.

In summary, CEOs, governing boards, and other members of a hospital's top management team should learn to think in terms of what is happening externally and how this affects the institution: new opportunities that are emerging and existing opportunities that may be declining, threats that jeopardize a hospital's well being or even its survival, barriers that may limit or reduce its capacity for service, the plans of its competitors that may disturb existing arrangements or markets, and the needs and expectations of the many groups that are affected by what management does, should do, or neglects to do. A key lies in distinguishing between external changes over which management has some control and those over which it has no control. Strategies can be devised to maneuver the hospital around emerging uncontrollable situations or to influence others who may be able to change these situations. Constant vigilance is required to monitor and assess the environment and weigh the impact of external change. When combined with an assessment of the institution's capabilities, its strengths, and its weaknesses, this knowledge provides the underpinnings for strategic thinking.

Notes

1. Rothschild, William E. *Putting It All Together: A Guide to Strategic Thinking.* New York City: AMACOM, 1976, p. 2.

2. Christopher, William F. *Management for the 1980s.* Englewood Cliffs, N.J.: Prentice-Hall, Inc., 1980, p. 134.

3. Steiner, George A., and Miner, John B. *Management Policy and Strategy.* New York City: Macmillan Publishing Co., Inc., 1977, p. 41.

4. See Foy, Nancy. *The Yin and Yang of Organizations.* New York City: William Morrow and Company, Inc., 1980, pp. 176-78. This reference includes an analysis of a model developed by John Morris at the Manchester Business School that is useful in understanding the kinds of activities carried out by management.

5. The environment of a business is likened to the environment of any other organic entity, an analogy that underscores the complexity of the various environmental forces that must be taken into account in developing a corporate strategy, in Andrews, Kenneth R. *The Concept of Corporate Strategy.* Homewood, IL: Richard D. Irwin, Inc., 1980, p. 48 ff.

6. McCarthy, Daniel J., and others. *Business Policy and Strategy: Concepts and Readings.* Homewood, IL: Richard D. Irwin, Inc., 1979, p. 178.

7. Health Central, Inc. *Strategic Challenges for the Eighties: An Environmental Assessment of the Health Care Industry in the Upper Midwest.* Paper prepared for owned, leased, and managed hospitals. Minneapolis, Jan. 1981, p. 3.

8. Tuller, Edwin, and Kozak, David. Logical thought process key to corporate plan. *Hospitals, J.A.H.A.* 53:82, Sept. 1, 1979.

9. National Center for Health Statistics. *Health Resources Statistics—Health Manpower and Health Facilities,* 1976-1977 edition. Washington, DC: DHEW, 1977, p. 415.

10. Ansoff, H. Igor. *Strategic Management.* New York City: John Wiley & Sons, 1981, pp. 186-87, and Managing surprise by response to weak signals. *California Management Review.* 18:21, Winter 1975.

11. Quinn, James Brian. Managing strategic change, *Sloan Management Review.* 21:3, Summer 1980. More than four centuries ago, Niccolo Machiavelli wrote in *The Prince,* chapter 3, ". . . for knowing afar off . . . the evils that are brewing, they are easily cured. But when, for want of such knowledge, they are allowed to grow until everyone can recognize them, there is no longer any remedy to be found."

12. Quinn, p. 3.

13. There are three prescriptive paperback guides, all in a lighthearted vein, that outline some easy-to-apply techniques for personal growth in dealing with the future and the problems that invariably accompany it: Kobert, Don, and Bagnall, Jim. *The Universal Traveller—A Soft-System Guide to Creativity, Problem-Solving and the Process of Reaching Goals.* Los Altos, CA: William Kaufmann, Inc., 1976; Bolles, Richard N. *The Three Boxes of Life—And How to Get Out of Them.* Berkeley, CA: Ten Speed Press, 1978; and Campbell, David. *If You Don't Know Where You're Going, You'll Probably End Up Somewhere Else.* Niles, IL: Argus Communications, 1974.

14. On developing issue statements, see Webber, James B., and Dula, Martha A. Effective planning committees for hospitals. *Harvard Business Review.* 52:133, May-June 1974; and Jordan, Margaret. *Discovering the Issues: A First Step in Plan Development.* Seattle, WA: Technical Assistance and Continuing Education Project, University of Washington, 1975.

15. Quoted in Ellis, Darryl J., and Pekar, Peter P. Jr. *Planning for Nonplanners.* New York City: AMACOM, 1980, p. 27.

16. Just as many nationally oriented publications such as *The New York Times, Washington Post, Business Week, Fortune, Time, Newsweek, and Harvard Business Review* provide ambitious executives with timely information on what is happening in the outside world to keep them ahead of change, many periodicals and newsletters inform health care professionals about happenings, trends, new ideas, and changes in the health care field. Each week the American Hospital Association publishes *Hospital Week,* a newsletter designed to expedite news items of particular interest to hospital management, and *Health Law Vigil,* a biweekly newsletter with a fast-track news service that analyzes legislative, regulatory, and judicial developments affecting hospitals.

    Several journals are helpful: *Hospitals* and *Trustee* magazines, published by American Hospital Publishing, Inc., Chicago; and *Modern Healthcare,* published by Crain Communications, Inc., Chicago; *Hospitals & Health Services Administration,* published by the American College of Hospital Administrators, Chicago; *Inquiry,* published by the Blue Cross Association; *Health Services Research,* published by the Hospital Research and Educational Trust, Chicago; *Health Care Management Review,* published by Aspen Systems, Corp., Germantown, MD; the *American Journal of Public Health,* published by Health Assoc., Washington, DC; and the *Milbank Memorial Fund Quarterly,* published by MIT Press, Cambridge, MA.

    For lay readers interested in current issues in medicine, the *New England Journal of Medicine,* published by the Massachusetts Medical Society, Boston, merits special attention. In addition, *The Futurist,* published by the World Future Society, Washington, DC, is an interesting magazine that specializes in matters that promise to affect future life-styles.

    For a list of journals, periodic reports, graduate programs, and organizations in futures research, see in Fowles, Jib, editor. *Handbook of Futures Research.* Westport, CT: Greenwood Press, 1978, appendix, pp. 803-6. For more detail, see *Resources Directory for America's Third Century.* Part II. *Information Sources for the Study of the Future.* Washington, DC: World Future Society, 1977. Several subscription services supply advice on various aspects of the future. Some are expensive, but apparently worth the price to satisfied clients. The Futures Group, Glastonbury, CT, issues *Prospects,* its consumer studies, and *Futurscan,* a document oriented to policy analysis. SRI International, Menlo Park, CA., provides clients with data from the scores of future studies that it conducts for businesses and governments worldwide. Yankelovich, Skelly, and White, Inc., New York City, offers a variety of survey services that alert others to the future consequences of events and trends in key areas of the nation.

17. Zentner, p. 50.

18. The use of environmental scanning is still in its infancy. As a result, no definite prescription can be given that is useful in all situations. See Fahey, Liam, and King, William R. Environmental scanning for corporate planning. *Business Horizons.* 20:61, Aug. 1977.

19. TAP was developed by the predecessor organization of the American Council of Life Insurance and depends on the efforts of volunteer monitors who work for the council's member companies. Each monitor regularly scans one or more publications for ideas or events that are indicative of trends or environmental discontinuities that have possible implications for the future concerns of society and the life insurance industry. The monitor also abstracts the possible significance to business. These abstracts are analyzed six times a year by a special in-house committee of the council's staff and less frequently by a steering committee of

senior officers from member companies. The results are circulated to the council's members. TEAM is a proprietary program produced by three former staff members of the American Council of Life Insurance, which formed the independent consulting firm Weiner, Edrich, Brown, Inc., to help business undertake a program similar to TAP. TEAM also relies on volunteer monitors and passes the results through the sieve of an oversight steering committee. For more information on TAP and TEAM, including the pros and cons of these approaches, see Brown, James K. *This Business of Issues: Coping with the Company's Environments.* Conference Board Report No. 758. New York City: The Conference Board, Inc., 1979, pp. 22-9.

For more on use of various tools in forming an organization's version of its present and future environment, see Zentner, Rene D. How to evaluate the present and future corporate environment. *The Journal of Business Strategy.* 1:42, Spring 1981.

20. William E. Rothschild presents a succinct, but enlightening analysis of the importance of stakeholders in determining an organization's strategy and objectives in *Putting It All Together: A Guide to Strategic Thinking.* New York City: AMACOM, 1976, pp. 188-95. For further applications, see Emshoff, James R., and Freeman, R. Edward. *Stakeholder Management.* Working Paper no. 3-78. Philadelphia: The Wharton Applied Research Center, Nov. 1978.

21. There are various sources for this figure. SRI International, Menlo Park, CA, first developed the concept in 1963.

22. Adapted in part from Rothschild, William E. Competitor analysis: the missing link in strategy. *Management Review.* 68:22, July 1979.

23. On the interrelationship between planning and seeking a competitive advantage, see Glueck, W. F., and others. Strategic management for competitive advantage. *Harvard Business Review.* 58:154, July-Aug. 1980; and South, Stephen E. Competitive advantage: the cornerstone of strategic thinking. *The Journal of Business Strategy.* Spring 1981.

24. Porter, Michael E. How competitive forces shape strategy. *Harvard Business Review.* 57:137, Mar.-Apr. 1979.

25. Rogatz, Peter. Directions of health system for a new decade. *Hospitals.* 54:67, Jan. 1, 1980.

26. Melum, Mara M. Hospitals must change, control is the issue. *Hospitals.* 54:67, Mar. 1, 1980.

27. Ellis and Pekar, p. 39.

28. See Peters, Joseph P. *A Guide to Strategic Planning for Hospitals.* Chicago: AHA, 1979, pp. 20-1; and American Hospital Association. *The Practice of Planning in Health Care Institutions.* Chicago: AHA, 1973, chapter 3 and appendixes B and C.

29. See Zimmerman, J. P. Service areas and their needs. *Hospitals, J.A.H.A.* 49:46, Sept. 1, 1975; and Greater Detroit Area Hospital Council, Inc. *Patient Origin and Hospital Use Studies.* Detroit: The Council.

30. Allio, Robert J., and Pennington, Malcolm W. *Corporate Planning, Techniques, and Applications,* New York City: AMACOM, 1979, pp. 8-9.

31. Glueck, W. F. *Strategic Management and Business Policy.* New York City: McGraw-Hill Book Company, 1980, pp. 116-17.

32. The authors were introduced to this concept in a presentation given by General Electric. However, it is now a well-known and widely used tool in industry.

Chapter 5
Introduction to Forecasting

"Virtually all decision making involves an element of forecasting. In making any choice which can be postponed, some type of forecast is involved, explicitly or implicitly, in order to decide on the best timing. Whenever the wisdom of a choice depends to some extent on future conditions, choosing implies forecasting. Forecasting, therefore, is an integral part of decentralized private decision making."

—Gerald Sirkin, *The Visible Hand: Fundamentals of Economic Planning*[1]

"Crystal balls in which we can see the economic future of an industry, let alone a nation, have been in short supply. Yet businessmen and governments must look to the future in formulating economic policies. They must predict; they always have, relying heavily on data, judgment, and intuition. During the last few years, however, *objective analytical* methods have come to play a major role in economic forecasting. Informed judgment is as important as ever, but the purely subjective elements are reduced."

—Victor Zarnowitz, *The New York Times*[2]

"But there is another kind of corporate planning. This consists of attempts to portray the aspects of the future that are of interest to management. Assumptions are made concerning trends which are not yet discernible, circumstances which have not yet crystallized, events which have not yet occurred, decisions which have not yet been reached."

—Dean E. Wooldbridge, *The Corporate Planning Process*[3]

Strategy is, by its very nature, concerned with the future, and this is perhaps a major reason why so few people are able to carry it out successfully. Many managers are harried with problems of the moment and push aside the uncertainties of tomorrow. Of course, sound epistemologic reasons exist for this preoccupation with the present. The present is the realm of all our perceptions and actions; in fact, acting or even existing in any other dimension but the here and now is impossible.

And yet, the future is perceptually an essential part of life. It is certainly the focus of much of our thoughts and actions. Of all created beings, humans alone have the capacity to determine their own future.[4] Indeed, all strategies and planning efforts are grounded in the belief that certain actions taken today will change the world that we will experience tomorrow. As Walter Firey of the University of Texas has so perceptively observed, "The theory of planning finds its subject matter in propositions which have their place in the future but which might not become real in the absence of the plan."[5] If humans did not possess this capacity to shape some aspects of the future, planning would be futile; we would be subject to the relentless forces of a totally predictable world.

Much of the world is, to be sure, totally predictable: the sun will rise and set and tides will change at predictable, precise times for all tomorrows, just as they have done in all the yesterdays that have passed. Some events under human control are equally predictable but can be changed, although with great difficulty; for example, April 15 is the income tax deadline in the United States, and Social Security checks are delivered on scheduled dates.

Five Basic Periods of Future Time

1. Now: The Immediate Future (up to one year from now)
   Prime characteristics:
   - Frozen/dictated by the past
   - Uncontrollable
   - Unlockable, except by a major event, usually a catastrophe
   - Present decisions or actions have little or no effect on this time frame
   - Minor choices available (what to wear, vacations, what to eat, and so forth)
2. Near-Term/Short-Term Futures (1 to 5 years)
   Prime characteristics:
   - Past-programmed future
   - Crisis-programmed change; incremental reactive change possible
   - Evolutionary advances become possible to be implemented
   - Partially controllable from today
   - Decisions made today can cause major shifts; major efforts are required to bring about revolutionary change
   - Policy choices are available: new programs, systems, institutions, and leaders may be initiated to cause impact
3. Middle-Range Futures (5 to 20 years)
   Prime characteristics:
   - Choice of alternative futures; choice available from alternative opportunities that the future offers, if awareness of alternatives exists in the present
   - Almost completely controllable and decidable today
   - Revolutionary change may be implemented from directed evolutionary (small) changes initiated today
   - Almost anything imaginable becomes possible to bring about
   - The future available in this time frame is inevitable and shapable today
   - Today's decisions can solidify this future time frame
4. Long-Range Futures (20 to 50 years hence)
   Prime characteristics:
   - Opportunities and/or crises triggerable/seedable today
   - Many alternative opportunities can be made visible
   - Open futures
5. Far Futures (50 years and beyond)
   Prime characteristics:
   - Largely invisible (to today)
   - Uncontrollable future (from today)
   - Utopian and dystopian speculation possible

—Reprinted, with permission, from
Earl C. Joseph, *An Introduction to the Study of Future*[6]

Yet much of the future, particularly those aspects that fall within the domain of strategic thinking, is unknown and always uncertain, and management must learn how to deal with these unknowns and uncertainties. This by no means implies, however, that the inherent epistemologic nonreality of the future and its resulting uncertainty prevent management from knowing the future or effectively confronting it. Humans are able to think in terms of what the future will look like and what it should look like. This ability is sufficient to enable management to cope with the future with more success than one might expect, given the complexity of this time dimension. Determining what the future will look like is called *forecasting* and deciding what it should look like is simply another phrase for *planning*. The two notions should not be confused. Planning is designed to *make* something happen; forecasting tells us what is *expected* to happen.[7]

Elements of Forecasting

Forecasting is a key ingredient in strategic thinking. Not only must management develop strategies for handling future uncertainties, but also it must recognize that the consequences of these strategies can extend far into the future. As a result, management must be able to deal with two unknowns: the emerging future and the possible consequences of current decisions in that future. *Both notions entail forecasting.*

Much has been written about forecasting and the various techniques for making forecasts. Despite the growing complexity of the subject, the essence of forecasting can be distilled into a simple how-to-do-it approach that is adaptable to most hospital managerial situations. Indeed, several good reasons exist for a simple approach:

- Many studies have shown that the increased accuracy of complex models is rarely worth the time and cost. Even relying on experts has been shown to be of little value once their expertise passes a certain minimal level.[8]
- Planners have discovered that if managers are unable to understand a forecasting model or an approach, they will not use it. In fact, highly sophisticated techniques often turn off management.
- Fancy techniques often become outdated and can be misused in widespread application, thus losing whatever advantages they may have.
- Matching the forecasting method to the situation being forecasted is more important than the elaboration of the technique.

Here are a few basic techniques that have proven helpful in carrying out the forecasting task. They separate this task into the various elements and assumptions that underlie it and identify the several choices that are required in making a forecast. More important, they emphasize the notion that forecasting for planning purposes is moving away from complexity toward simplicity.

Every forecast consists of two elements: the *current status* of the situation or variable and its future change. Most persons pay little attention to the former, not realizing that many forecasting errors are caused by failure to define the current status or starting point. Dividing the forecasting problem into an analysis of current status and future change can alert the forecaster to potential difficulties.[9] Abraham Lincoln gave some good advice on this matter: "If we could first know where we are and whither we are tending, we could then better judge what to do and how to do it." A good rule to follow is *expend as much effort in measuring current status as in forecasting future change.*

Determining the current status of a situation is the basic building block for a forecast. For example, in forecasting its future share of a local market, a hospital first must determine its present share of that market and also must understand the various factors that contribute to or limit its market share. Likewise, the accuracy of a population forecast for a given area may be questionable either because the count of the present population is not accurate or the count itself is a projection based on limited or inaccurate facts. If the population of a hospital's service area or market is projected to increase at one percent per year for the next decade, it can make a great difference if its present population is estimated at 92,000 rather than 110,000. In intercensal periods, current estimates for small areas such as hospital markets are often imprecise. A 10 percent error in either direction may invalidate even the most sophisticated forecast.

The forecasting task can be approached as a *series of choices,* organized as follows: choices com mon to all forecasting tasks, choices of core assumptions underlying the forecast, and choices of the forecasting technique.[10]

The first set of choices, those common to all forecasting tasks, is concerned with the components of the task itself. These choices focus on such questions as the following: Who will make the forecast and using what methods? Should management make its own forecasts or use a consensus of existing forecasts? Should management purchase forecasts from one of the many organizations marketing such services? How many judgmental adjustments are necessary and at what points should they be made in the forecasting process? Should the forecast be limited to isolated trends such as competition in the health care field, or be broadened to include all interrelated factors such as the economic, political, legal, and market forces that could spur increasing competition? Here, the trick is, of course, to determine what will work best in one's own situation and then to do it.

The second set of choices, those of core assumptions that support the forecast, is a key element in forecasting. Therefore, much of what follows in this chapter is an elaboration of this subject. The third set, choices of forecasting methods, involves the particular methods most appropriate and most applicable to the organization's capabilities and circumstances.

More about Making Core Assumptions

> "If enough questions begin with the word *why* and if they are posed in a chain or series, a distillation of purpose begins to appear. That distilled purpose is the definition as it is envisioned by the problem solver who asks and answers the questions. The why-chain is a boiling-down process. It forces a constant clarification of objectives until an accepted essence statement is reached.
>
> "Try not to stop until at least 10 'why' questions have been answered, and remember that it is better to be a whys-guy than never to have learned at all."
> —Don Koberg and Jim Bagnall,
> *The Universal Traveller*[11]

The second and third sets of choices incorporate interrelated assumptions, core assumptions about the future and theoretical assumptions underlying the projection technique. The core assumptions behind a forecast reflect the forecaster's basic outlook on the context within which the specific forecasted happening or trend develops. They include the background conditions, relationships, and basic trends that guide the preparation of a forecast. In the health care field, examples of core assumptions are the belief that the fee-for-service principle will continue to govern future payments for medical services, that the general hospital will continue to serve as the hub of the health care system, or that nursing will remain essentially a profession for women who will usually prepare for it when they complete high school. Obviously, if these assumptions prove to be unwarranted, forecasts about future patterns of financing medical care, the role of the hospital in tomorrow's society, or future nursing resources may also prove to be inaccurate. William Ascher found that the core assumptions in a forecast, not the choice of methodology, are the major determinants of forecast accuracy.[12] Thus, a basic piece of advice can be given to managers: *spend more time preparing and evaluating the assumptions on which subsequent forecasts will be made than worrying about the potential accuracy of a given technique.* The best techniques cannot save a forecast that is built on unsubstantiated or questionable assumptions.

Forecasting for health care services, unlike other types of forecasting such as predicting the weather, involves assumptions about human and organizational behavior. These assumptions include a hospital's service area and changes in that area, the behavior of physicians and patients, the competitive interaction of different types of health care providers, the rate of technological innovation, the economic climate, the political and regulatory environment (what happens if P.L. 93-641 is not extended), changing values of society, and other basic matters. For example, a prevailing assumption made by many hospitals is that health maintenance organizations will cut into their market and affect their census and the type of patients they treat. Thus, a review of core assumptions in a forecast for the health care field should question what assumptions about human behavior or about societal changes the forecasters have included. A few other questions should be asked when testing core assumptions:

- What objective evidence or experiments have been generated to solve the problem at hand?
- What objective evidence or empirical studies have been developed by others?
- How much subjective evidence from unbiased outside experts such as consultants or technical papers is contained in the assumption?
- Is the assumption based mainly on subjective impressions of persons within the organization?

Once the core assumptions have been made and the forecaster is satisfied with their validity, the next step involves selecting an appropriate technique for forecasting the future based on these assumptions.

Some general comments about forecasting techniques are needed. A distinction exists between techniques used to predict the future and other tools employed by forecasters. For example, extrapolation—extending historical data into the future on the assumption that the future will conform to the past—is a familiar forecasting technique. Cross-impact analysis—a technique based on the concept that events are linked and that the occurrence of an event affects the likelihood that other events will follow—is a tool used by forecasters to modify or sharpen an extrapolation.[13] Econometric modeling is another forecasting technique, whereas scenario writing is a way of examining various possibilities rather than of making forecasts.

All of these techniques reflect a trend away from relying on subjective methods such as judgment and intuition to the use of well-specified, objective processes that translate statistical and other inputs into forecasts that can be replicated by other forecasters. However, subjective, judgmental approaches are appropriate in some instances. The success of various judgmental techniques such as interviews, questionnaires, Delphi, and nominal group process in soliciting ideas on future happenings attests to their usefulness.

Delphi Forecasting

The Delphi Technique is a method of forecasting social and organizational futures by obtaining consensus from a panel of experts on the probability that certain events will occur. The technique is simple, although it entails considerable structuring and feedback. A panel of knowledgeable persons who remain anonymous and whose participation is not made known to the other members is organized to monitor given subjects. A questionnaire is developed to solicit the panelists' assessments/predictions on selected subjects or themes. The returns are processed and used to develop a second questionnaire; as many additional responses and questionnaires are circulated as are required to reach a consensus on anticipated future changes. Delphi is especially useful in complex situations that do not lend themselves to precise analytical techniques but that can benefit from collective subjective judgments by knowledgeable persons who are not constrained by face-to-face exchanges.[14]

Extrapolation and econometric approaches are becoming increasingly popular, despite the difficulty in weaning persons away from judgmental methods.[15] Extrapolation is a general term for a variety of objective forecasting techniques used for determining future values of a variable based on historical patterns. Specific techniques include trend projection, time series analysis, and regression analysis. Econometric approaches are objective, causal methods based on regression analysis. They project the future by using causal relationships.[16] In some instances, econometrics can transcend extrapolations to explain the sources of uncertainty.

Extrapolation and econometric approaches have an additional advantage over subjective methods in that it is easier to save data to allow for a simulation of the forecasts. They also provide an explicit record for future use, and the results can be replicated by other forecasters.

Finally, when changes are large, as in long-range forecasting, the forecasting method must contribute to learning. Extrapolation methods are of little value in this respect, but econometric methods can be very helpful. However, most persons have great confidence in their ability to use judgmental forecasting methods and to learn from them. This confidence is completely unfounded, as the unaided judge is an inefficient learner. The basic reason is that a person rarely uses disconfirming evidence. The problem is especially serious for those who view themselves as experts. Many of them continue to use the same model, even when conditions change.

Advice on Preparing and Using Forecasts

J. Scott Armstrong has formulated 17 tough questions that management should consider in carrying out a forecasting effort. Here is a summary of his key thoughts:

- Eliminate top management from direct involvement in actual forecasting tasks. Management is likely to be biased toward an overly optimistic view of the future.
- Don't rely on any single forecasting method. Be eclectic.
- Keep it simple. Use methods that can be understood by the user.
- Don't listen to persons such as Henry Ford who believe that "history is bunk." Use historical data in a systematic way to overcome the tendency of experts to rely too heavily on the latest information.
- The plan, not the forecast, should motivate management action. "If the forecast is not satisfactory to management, they should change the plan, not the forecast—that would be like changing the weather forecast to make your picnic a success."
- There is a point of diminishing returns in accumulating information. Rather than allocating more time and money to the search for more information, make better use of the information already available.
- Beware of ignoring forecasts that contradict management's prior beliefs or expectations.
- Use this four-step procedure to evaluate your forecasting task:
  1. Assess the process, not the forecast.
  2. Examine the assumptions and data supporting the forecast.
  3. Specify and contest the uncertainties that are part of any forecast.
  4. Weigh the costs of the forecast.

—Summarized from J. Scott Armstrong, *Directors and Boards*[17]

Appraising a Forecast

Forecasting is as much an art as it is a science. There are many techniques that can be used in carrying out the forecasting task, each with its particular strength and limitations. It is, therefore, appropriate that a forecast be evaluated in terms of questions such as these:[18]

- What is being forecast?
- Does the forecast show current status and future changes?
- What are the core assumptions that form the basis of the forecast? Are they plausible? What is the sensitivity of the forecast to changes in one or more of the core assumptions? These questions can be answered by looking for:
  —Background forecasts used in the preparation of this forecast
  —Both explicit and implicit assumptions about trends and relationships
  —Assumptions about basic human behavior
  —Objective and subjective sources of evidence behind the assumptions
  —"Assumption drag," the reliance on out-of-date core assumptions
- What technique(s) were used in the forecast?
  —Were they subjective or objective?
  —If objective, were they extrapolations or causal models?
  —Are the methods acceptable to the users?
  —Does the logical structure of the method fit the situation?
  —Does the method fit the purpose of the forecast, for example, do assessing the uncertainty of a decision and assessing alternative futures contribute to learning?
  —Do the forecasting method and the situation match to produce the best possible level of accuracy?
- Are there sources of bias in the forecaster's characteristics, the institutional base, or training and specialization?
- In application of judgment to the forecast, is there evidence of bias among the judges, such as the tendency to confuse their desires with their forecasts, or of anchoring, the tendency for judges to be conservative and bound by tradition?
- Have the forecasters done the best job they can to include sociopolitical factors that might influence the results?

Although forecasting is never an easy task, it need not be complicated. As already noted, the task involves two steps: an analysis of the current status of the situation and then a forecast of future changes by blending valid core assumptions with an appropriate forecasting method. And a good forecaster must always be prepared to revise both the assumptions and the forecast as conditions change or as new evidence is brought to bear on the situation.

Notes

1. Sirkin, Gerald. *The Visible Hand: The Fundamentals of Economic Planning.* New York City: McGraw-Hill, Inc., 1968, p. 49.
2. Zarnowitz, Victor. University of Chicago. In: *The New York Times.* 30:447, Oct. 26, 1980.
3. Wooldbridge, Dean E. Introduction. In: Branch, Melville C. *The Corporate Planning Process.* New York City: American Management Association, 1962, p. 14.
4. For further elaboration on the nature of the future and humans' ability to shape it, see World Future Society. *An Introduction to the Study of the Future.* Washington, DC: The Society, 1977, chapter 6; de Jouvenel, Bertrand. *The Art of Conjecture.* New York City: Basic Books, Inc. Publishers, 1967; Fowles, Jib, editor. *Handbook of Futures Research.* Westport, CT: Greenwood Press, 1978, part 2; and Ozbekhan, Hasan. Toward a general theory of planning. In: Jantsch, Erich. *Perspectives of Planning.* Paris: Organisation for Economic Co-operation and Development, 1968.
5. Firey, Walter. *Law and Economy in Planning.* Austin, TX: University of Texas Press, 1965, p. 5.
6. Joseph, Earl C. In: World Future Society. *An Introduction to the Study of the Future.* Washington, DC: The Society, 1977, pp. 131-32.
7. For more information on this distinction, see Armstrong, J. Scott. *Long-Range Forecasting: From Crystal Ball to Computer.* New York City: John Wiley & Sons, 1978, pp. 5-7.
8. Armstrong, pp. 84-6.
9. Armstrong, p. 53 ff.
10. This outline of the forecasting task is adapted from Ascher, William. *Forecasting: An Appraisal for Policy Makers and Planners.* Baltimore: The Johns Hopkins Press, 1978.
11. Koberg, Don, and Bagnall, Jim. *The Universal Traveller: A Soft-Systems Guide to Creativity, Problem-Solving and the Process of Reaching Goals.* Los Altos, CA: William Kaufmann, Inc., 1976, p. 62.
12. Ascher, p. 199.
13. For an elaboration on the uses of cross-impact analysis, see Stover, John G., and Gordon, Theodore J. Cross-impact analysis. In: Fowles, Jib, editor. *Handbook of Futures Research.* Westport, CT: Greenwood Press, 1978.
14. For more information on general applications of Delphi, see Linstone, Harold A. The Delphi Technique. In: Fowles, Jib, editor. Handbook of Futures Research. Westport, CT: Greenwood Press, 1978, pp. 273-300; for health services applications, see Spiegel, Allen D., and Hyman, Herbert Harvey. *Basic Health Planning Methods.* Germantown, MD: Aspen Systems Corporation, 1978, pp. 49-51, 160-1.
15. Armstrong, chapter 16.
16. Armstrong, chapter 7.
17. A summary of ideas provided in Armstrong, J. Scott. What to ask about management's forecast: seventeen tough questions. *Directors and Boards.* 6:20, Summer 1981.
18. Based on ideas from Armstrong and Ascher.

Chapter 6

Conducting an Internal Analysis

"The internal analysis by itself reveals much about where the company has been (or what it has been doing) and where it is now (or what it now is doing). It should also reveal something about the ways in which the future is being approached. . . . Combining an internal and external analysis will produce the complete assessment which will allow the analyst . . . to see not only what the organization is capable of doing in light of its resources, but often what it ought to be doing considering the external environment in which it operates."

—Daniel J. McCarthy and others,
Business Policy and Strategy: Concepts and Readings[1]

"Seek out some of the 'dirty jobs' in analysis. Truth often hides in corners."

—Don Koberg and Jim Bagnall,
The Universal Traveller: A Soft-Systems Guide to Creativity, Problem-Solving and the Process of Reaching Goals[2]

"The individual often has trouble knowing himself: where he came from, how he got where he is, what he must do next to survive, to grow, to be a useful member of society.

"Similarly, an organization may have difficulty defining its strengths, setting specific goals, and charting the paths to reach them. . . . In time, the need for a formal review of both the program and its operations—of goals and how to reach them—becomes evident. That time is hastened by the acquisition of new leadership and an appreciation of the growing complexity of the constantly changing world."

—The Rockefeller Foundation,
The Course Ahead: The Rockefeller Foundation in the Next Five Years[3]

An enterprise must be alert to what is happening in the outside world and how these external events may affect its operations, but it must also take steps to *know itself* if it hopes to manage the opportunities and threats that the outside world brings to it. To do this, it must identify its strengths, which enable it to accomplish the things it sets out to do, and uncover its weaknesses, which limit its ability to accomplish things.

Never an easy task and often distasteful, an internal analysis forces management to focus its attention on what the organization has done in the past and what it is doing now; how well it is presently performing; what it is capable or incapable of doing given its present structure, resources, strategy, and values; where it is headed if it continues business as usual; and whether it has the capabilities to deal with the uncertainties of the future.

When done honestly and perceptively, an internal analysis enables an organization to achieve a high degree of self-awareness that is so important to survival and growth in turbulent times. Indeed, devising a strategy for the future can be likened to making arrangements for a journey. Without the appropriate resources, an alert leadership, and a shared sense of direction, an organization can expect to face the same hazards in the uncertain world of tomorrow that an unprepared person lacking the essential gear or a good map is likely to face on a long voyage to an unfamiliar land. When an organization's or person's resources, abilities, and values are mismatched to new circumstances and opportunities, everything else seems unimportant.[4]

Procedures for Self-Assessment

Through frank, open discussion, examine the institution's strengths and weaknesses in terms of where it has been, where it is today, and where it is headed.

Bring to bear as much objective information as possible, such as employee turnover ratios, insurance surveys, and outside accreditation and licensing reports, and augment existing information sources by special studies.

Challenge all statements about the hospital's accomplishments and capabilities, question the relevancy of its programs, evaluate the adequacy of its resources, appraise the quality of its services, examine reasons for past success and for past failures, and project where the institution is headed if it continues business as usual.

Be hard-nosed in your assessments! Don't be afraid to ask, "Who said so?" or "Why must this be so?" or "Can we do what we are doing better?" Ask probing questions.

Review all activities and ask, "If the organization were not committed to the activity at the present time, would it initiate it today?" If the answer is no, it may be wise to abandon the activity as quickly as possible.

Be open to bad news and complaints.

Don't ever assume that all is well within the hospital. Most especially, don't fall victim to your own public relations!

Don't be defensive. Peter Drucker warns that unless management is prepared to carry out an honest probe of what's happening both inside and outside the organization, it will waste its energy defending yesterday and no one will have the urge to work on exploiting today, let alone to work on creating a desired future.

Keep in mind that a successful past can be positively dangerous if it leaves management content with the present and ill-equipped to meet tomorrow's demands.

A logical starting point in conducting an internal analysis to determine an organization's capacity to adjust to its environment is the organization's present strategy and its success in applying it (see the questions listed in chapter 3). However, because many hospitals do not have a formal strategy to which they can readily refer, they should follow Norman McMillan's advice, "Start . . . by digging out the facts about your hospital."[5] But what hospital activities should be included in this assessment? "The total entity and everything in and around it," according to experts on business strategy.[6] Of course, within each area there are almost limitless elements and activities that can be scrutinized (see figure 10, Internal Areas to Be Analyzed in Assessing Strengths and Weaknesses of a Hospital).

The following discussion focuses on some major areas to be included in any assessment, with a simple

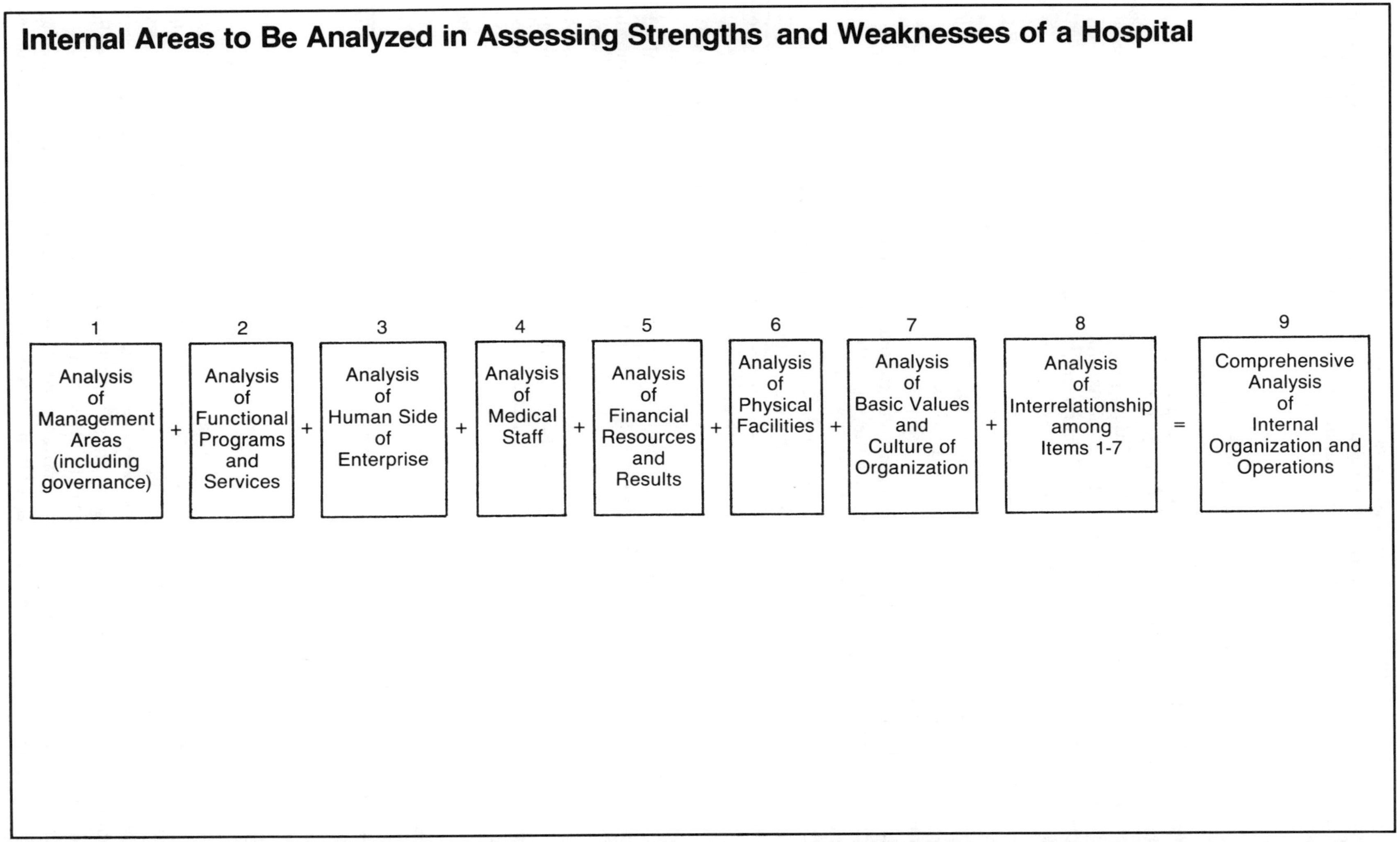

Figure 10. These eight major areas should be included in any comprehensive analysis of an organization's internal operations.[7]

list of the types of questions to be asked and factors to be studied in each area. Neither the list nor the questions are all-inclusive. However, they should provide sufficient clues for conducting a meaningful, in-depth internal assessment. For example, *management and governance* is as good an area as any in which to commence an internal analysis. The following questions are helpful in examining top management and what it does:

- What person or group is really in charge and is this known throughout the organization? How does this affect what goes on within the organization?
- What are the role and contributions of the governing board? Do its members know what they are supposed to do, and are they aware of their responsibilities? Is the board effective in guiding the affairs of the institution? How are its members selected? Is it a working body? Is there sufficient turnover to encourage new ideas?
- What is the overall quality and reputation of management? Does it deliver what is expected of it by the board, medical staff, employees, patients, and other stakeholders? What has it neglected to do? How does management spend its time?
- Is management prepared to meet the challenges of the future? Is it prepared to handle unexpected "what if" situations? Is it committed to and capable of carrying out a meaningful long-range planning effort that results in desired actions?
- Is management making an effort to retain its vigor, to recruit new staff into its ranks, to encourage middle managers and department heads to acquire new skills and broaden their perspectives? Are managers interested in keeping abreast of developments in the hospital industry? Do they keep their fingers on the pulse of the community?
- Does management have the courage to take calculated risks? Does it spend its time defending the past or the status quo? Is it capable of thinking in strategic terms?

The core of any internal assessment, of course, is *what the institution does*—its functions and programs, their scope and volume—and *how well it does what it does*—the quality of its services and products, patient satisfaction, and the institution's contributions to the health and welfare of its community. An enormous amount of statistical and other information useful in making such determinations is available within every hospital. Much of this information is regularly gathered for internal administrative, budgeting, and reporting purposes. A key determinant in how much information will be made available to the strategy management group is the expectations of the participants. Some hospital board members are accustomed to receiving detailed reports in their businesses or professions and often rely on computers to give these to them. Such members of a strategy management group can make heavy demands on staff for information, and staff should be prepared to meet these demands.[8]

The following questions should be raised and answered in evaluating various functions and programs within the hospital:

- What are we doing now?
- Why are we doing it?
- Are we doing it well?
- Can we do it better?
- Should we be doing it at all?
- Do other ways of doing it exist?
- How much is it costing us?
- Should we abandon the activity?

The utilization of the hospital's patient care services is an important barometer to understanding what is going on within the institution. Thus, many strategic discussions open with consideration of such matters as a decline in admissions, patient days, or occupancy rates; unexpected shifts in obstetrics-gynecology or pediatrics admissions; or some other development in the use of various patient care or diagnostic services. Information on these matters is usually collected on a regular basis by the hospital's medical records department and can be made available on short notice.

Because the *human element* is a factor in everything that a hospital does and how well it does it, this area should be analyzed independently, apart from other considerations. "The reality of organization behavior and human relations so influences the nature of . . . [an] organization that it must be considered as a major focus for the internal analysis. . . . If an organization can be judged to be 'healthy,' however, management has done much of its job, and the crucial human resources of the firm are probably a major asset to the organization.''[9]

Many aspects must be considered and many questions asked in assessing this vital human element. Here are some of the more obvious questions:

- Does the hospital encounter any unusual difficulties in recruiting and retaining personnel? Is it considered a good place to work? Do its salaries, fringe benefits, opportunities, and working conditions compare favorably with other local hospitals and businesses?
- Have clear and equitable personnel policies and practices been established? How are they communicated throughout the organization? Do they seem to be acceptable to the employees?
- Is morale a problem anywhere within the institution? If morale does not seem to be a problem, how can management verify this?
- Is management capable of promoting harmony throughout the organization? Is management viewed with suspicion? Are its orders, policies, and practices carried out grudgingly or not at all?
- What is the overall employee turnover rate? How does it compare with other local hospitals and businesses? Do any departments or groups experience a higher or lower turnover? What steps has management recently taken to limit or promote employee turnover?
- Does the hospital provide appropriate orientation programs and ample continuing education activities for its employees? Does it offer career development opportunities? Are employees taking advantage of these opportunities?
- How does the institution react to unions and other collective bargaining efforts? Is there any evidence that future problems may develop?
- Do informal networks or cliques work against the organization or promote self-serving groups or professional interests to the detriment of the organization?
- What is the overall climate of the organization? Do employees seem to work together to achieve organizational and departmental goals? Do employees appear to know what is going on in the institution? How does management know this?
- Are employees worried about the organization's future? Does management keep them informed about its strategies and long-range plans? Will the employees support a new strategy?

The role and contributions of a *medical staff* in a hospital are well known. Although physicians and other members of the healing professions are part of the overall human resources that comprise the internal organization of a hospital, they should be evaluated independently. Hospitals are learning that they must be alert to the natural selection that occurs among members of their medical staffs. Physicians retire or relocate to other communities, new physicians are attracted or recruited, some members qualify for new appointments or additional privileges by meeting specialty board requirements or through continuing education programs, others lose interest or enthusiasm and contribute less to the institution, and a few linger on, at times to the detriment of the organization. These are just some of the changes that affect the size, quality, and contributions of a hospital's medical staff and, in turn, the attractiveness and drawing power of the institution.

When a hospital takes a hard look at itself, its first conclusions often center on its medical staff: size, composition, age, individual admitting practices, personalities, need for additional specialty representations, or recruitment problems.[10] The following complaints often surface when a hospital conducts an internal assessment, particularly when members of the attending staff are asked to participate: ''Too many doctors will be retiring soon,'' ''The hospital's biggest admitter is leaving,'' ''We're not getting our share of general practitioners to refer patients to our specialists,'' or ''We are replacing the retiring physicians with young physicians who don't have the same sense of loyalty and who don't want to work as hard.'' The point is that a hospital's medical staff is a major resource that must be taken into account in developing a strategy for the future. A hospital must build around whatever strengths it possesses in terms of the present or future size and composition of its medical staff and that staff's willingness to support the work of the institution. A hospital can hardly expect to diversify its activities, add new programs, or expand its scope of services without a sufficient physician base on which to structure these efforts. Understanding what is happening among the medical staff is an important element in strategic thinking; indeed, it is extremely doubtful that any hospital CEO would ever forget to include it in such an assessment.

Financing is another essential, some would even claim that it is the most essential element in the success or failure of an enterprise, even to a hospital whose overall goals are generally more oriented to community service than to profit-making. Not only is it important to gain insight into the organization's overall financial situation, such as its assets and liabilities, fiscal soundness, and continuing ability to withstand recessions, inflation, and other economic forces, but it is also necessary to understand the flow of income and expenses that enables the institution to stay in business, meet its obligations, finance new ventures, replace worn out or obsolete equipment, and build reserves for future contingencies. Financial information supplies basic insights to the ability of an organization to withstand future shocks and meet new opportunities and challenges.

The following questions can provide guidance in this area:[11]

- What is the hospital's recent financial history? Has it been able to attract or develop the financial resources necessary to enable it to meet its operating goals and requirements?
- What percentage of its revenue is derived from the Medicare and Medicaid programs or other programs that pay on the basis of allowable cost rather than established charges?
- What costs and other financial requirements are or are not provided for other significant third-party reimbursement programs at the institution?
- What is the present legislative environment in your state regarding rate regulation or other matters that could affect the hospital's revenue? How would the hospital meet its financial needs under any pending legislation?
- What sources or plan does the hospital have to recover that portion of its costs that is not paid for by third parties?
- Does the hospital's cash flow enable it to meet its operating requirements promptly?
- Is the hospital actively pursuing philanthropic and other nonpatient sources of revenue? What does the future hold in this area?
- How does the service population mix and economic character of the hospital's market area affect its revenue and its contractual allowances?
- Does the hospital prepare a budget? Is it using flexible operating budget techniques? Do its budgeted rates include provisions for an operating margin to cover working capital needs, other facility and equipment requirements, and contingencies?
- Is capital available to meet projected future needs? Will it be available as long as needed, or can it be easily replaced?
- Does the hospital have a long-range plan for covering its debt-financing needs? Can existing loans be prepaid or extended?
- Does the institution have the financial and other resources to survive indefinitely as an independent institution?

Sooner or later in any strategic management effort, consideration must be given to the hospital's *physical facilities.* Buildings and facilities are the *bridge* that permits the person seeking health care and the physician and other health workers supplying that care to meet and make effective use of the necessary equipment and technology that neither can provide nor achieve independently.[12] Even though facilities are merely means and not ends in the provision of certain health services, it is difficult to visualize a hospital independent of the buildings it occupies.

A well-designed, well-constructed, well-equipped, and well-maintained plant is a key determinant in supplying safe and good hospital care. Conversely, an obsolete, poorly designed, cramped, or in other ways inadequate plant can impose serious constraints on what takes place within its walls. Therefore, whenever a hospital reviews its strategy or proposes a new strategy, it must give serious consideration to the capacity or usability of its facilities to house what is contemplated or to support the new strategy.

Most hospitals have an experienced architect or engineer to evaluate their existing facilities. Indeed, "Existing facilities constitute a resource whose value and best future use may well be subject to considerable debate. Objective evaluations by outside professionals cognizant of modern trends and who know or have been informed of the long-term future form a sound and necessary base for all future planning."[13] The findings are useful not only in assessing the plant's capabilities and limitations, its strengths and weaknesses, but also in enabling management to determine the institution's future facility requirements in meeting changing community needs or in carrying out a new strategy.

Although more will be said about them in another chapter, *values, beliefs, and the overall culture or climate of an organization* influence everything that the organization does or proposes to do. This influence is particularly evident in hospitals where long traditions and stern value systems form the basis of virtually every function and activity.

As for every human institution, hospitals have a spirit. This spirit has changed over the years from early charitable enterprises that supplied more compassion than cure to the present centers of scientific humanism where modern medicine, technology, and social welfare meet to serve the needs of the sick and injured. However, the basic human service orientation has not been lost. In each hospital, physicians, nurses, technicians, aides, managers, volunteers, and other support workers share a sense of dedicated concern, often unexpressed and perhaps not even realized, that enables them to work harmoniously in meeting the needs of patients. When well managed and coordinated, these values and motivations can be considerable strengths on which to build an institution's future. But they can also be major deterrents that must be overcome or minimized when they discourage innovation or limit new ventures. To ignore them in any strategic assessment is to flirt with failure.

Strong or Weak Compared to What?

Analyzing an institution's strengths and weaknesses is essentially a task of comparing its capabilities, resources, and activities with some self-selected or externally imposed standards and criteria. An institution can appraise itself in relation to its competitors, to its conformance to the standards or requirements of Joint Commission on Accreditation of Hospitals (JCAH), state licensing agencies, various professional societies, and other outside accrediting or regulatory agencies, to its own expectations of what ought to be, and to its own past performance. Data information systems also exist to which it can subscribe and which enable it to make some of these comparisons.[14]

In analyzing the various internal areas of activity, much information will be compiled on specific strenghths and weaknesses and how these can enhance or limit the institution's future. But even this is not enough. These findings merely describe the anatomy of the organization. To obtain a more comprehensive perspective and appreciation of what is taking place within the organization, management must understand how the various activities are interrelated, how they affect each other, how they form a totality capable of accomplishing the organization's mission and goals, and how they contribute to the public's perception of the image of the institution. In short, the findings must be organized in a meaningful profile that summarized the overall health of the organization and its capacity to cope successfully with outside change.

A useful technique in matching an institution's functional, managerial, and other resources and values, particularly its strengths and basic underpinnings, to its environment is to list these strengths in one column and the threats expected to occur within 5 to 10 years in another column (see figure 8, Vulnerability Analysis, chapter 4). The information in the two columns is matched to determine whether any of the institution's basic strengths and supports are threatened by expected future events. If so, corrective or avertive action may be required. Similarly, its weaknesses should also be matched with outside development to determine the institution's vulnerability to outside forces.

In short, evaluating the internal strengths and weaknesses of an institution is an essential element in handling outside opportunities and threats.[15] When the internal conditions and environment changes are matched, the institution is ready to move ahead to develop a strategy for the future.

A Large Midwest Hospital Examines Itself

As part of its efforts to give corporate direction to its board, medical staff, and support staff, a large Midwest hospital of more than 600 beds, with a long record of sophisticated long-range planning, carried out an institutional analysis. It compared its present position with where it had been five years earlier. The following summary lists its self-perceived strengths and weaknesses:

Strengths

The hospital has:

- Strengthened the overall medical staff in numbers and disciplines
- Replaced bed and support obsolete facilities
- Strengthened its private ambulatory services capability
- Damatically improved the hospital's financial position
- Improved overall census and program utilization profiles
- Increased the number of participants and scope of both inpatient and ambulatory services provided in the renal disease program
- Significantly increased utilization of the rehabilitation center
- Made inroads in both utilization and medical management of the burn unit
- Achieved high visibility and community acceptance of family-centered obstetrics services
- Replaced obsolete radiation therapy facilities and established a dedicated oncology unit
- Achieved high utilization in the extended care facility, including a strong profile of long-term private residents
- Established modern G.I. and cardiopulmonary laboratories and updated nuclear medicine, ultrasound, and echocardiography services
- Achieved a high level of trustee knowledge and participation
- Achieved a high level of visibility among the administrative team, both locally and nationally
- Achieved a high level of philanthropic support
- Achieved a reputation as being progressive and innovative
- Achieved a better patient mix from within its local market
- Increased the number and held constant in the percentage of patients from south of the interstate expressway
- Achieved a number two position (1979 Hospital Council Statistics) or higher among the three largest metropolitan hospitals in usage of emergency department, obstetrics, gynecology, and newborn services; and extended care
- Achieved a perceived position of number two or higher among the three largest metropolitan hospitals in the provision of cancer, cardiology, trauma, and alcohol treatment and alternate birthing services
- Achieved high standing with the regulatory agencies based on level of participation and positions taken
- Developed a network of satellite physicians' buildings

Weaknesses

The hospital has:

- Significant manpower shortages, especially among nurses, and problems of annual turnover and employee attitude
- Problems with declining inpatient and ambulatory surgery activities
- Not improved its position in a number of tertiary medical services, including specialized surgery, neurological services, and services for the aged
- Not improved its overall uncompensated care position
- Not improved its overall position in terms of community perception
- Not provided additional on-site physician office space
- Not developed a comprehensive marketing outreach program
- Not developed an integrated patient/public/staff education program
- Not been able, during the past two years, to recruit the number of new physicians into the complex that either of the two other large local hospitals have
- Not improved its inpatient market share position

Notes

1. McCarthy, Daniel J., and others. *Business Policy and Strategy: Concepts and Readings.* Homewood, IL: Richard D. Irwin, Inc., 1979, p. 107.

2. Koberg, Don, and Bagnall, Jim. *The Universal Traveller: A Soft-Systems Guide to Creativity, Problem-Solving and the Process of Reaching Goals.* Los Altos, CA: William Kaufman, 1976, p. 53.

3. The Rockefeller Foundation. The Course Ahead: The Rockefeller Foundation in the Next Five Years. Paper published by the Rockefeller Foundation, May 1974.

4. For a stimulating, easy-to-follow elaboration of this notion, see Koberg and Bagnall.

5. McMillan, Norman H. *Planning for Survival: A Handbook for Hospital Trustees.* Chicago: American Hospital Association, 1976, p. 37.

6. McCarthy and others, p. 111.

7. An adaptation and expansion of schema by McCarthy and others, p. 113.

8. Peters, Joseph P. *A Guide to Strategic Planning for Hospitals.* Chicago: American Hospital Association, 1979, chapter 2.

9. McCarthy and others, p. 129.

10. For some easy-to-apply matrixes in studying a hospital's medical staff, see McMillan, pp. 60-3.

11. Adapted from American Hospital Association, in collaboration with the Hospital Research and Educational Trust. *Hospital Trustee Development Program.* vol. 1. Chicago: AHA, 1979, topic 4, Financial Affairs.

12. This analogy of facilities as a bridge to effective health care is taken from National Commission on Community Health Services. *Health Care Facilities: The Community Bridge to Effective Health Services.* Washington, DC: Public Affairs Press, 1967.

13. Hardy, Owen B., and Lammers, Lawrence P. *Hospitals: The Planning and Design Process.* Germantown, MD: Aspen Systems Corporation, 1977, p. 72. For more on evaluating a hospital facility, see *Methods for Assessing Facility Modernization Pressures.* Madison, WI: Institute for Health Planning, Aug. 1981.

14. Some examples are Professional Activity Study (PAS), conducted by the Commission on Professional and Hospital Activities, Ann Arbor, MI; MONITREND for Hospitals and Program for Institutional Effectiveness Review (PIER), both available from the AHA; and such state arrangements as the Oklahoma Data Information System (ODIS), compiled by the Oklahoma Hospital Association, Tulsa, OK.

15. For additional readings on internal evaluation, see Stevenson, Howard H. Analyzing corporate strengths and weaknesses. Adapted from an essay in *Sloan Management Review.* 17:51, Spring 1976, and reprinted in Glueck, William F. *Strategic Management and Business Policy.* New York City: McGraw-Hill Book Company, 1980, pp. 186-95; Buchele, Robert B. How to evaluate a firm. *California Management Review.* 5:5, Fall 1962; Andrews, Kenneth R. *The Concept of Corporate Strategy.* Homewood, IL: Richard D. Irwin, Inc., 1980, chapter 3; and Hussey, David E. The corporated appraisal: assessing company strengths and weaknesses. In: Jain, S. and Singhvi, S., editors. *Essentials of Corporate Planning.* Oxford, OH: The Planning Executives Institute, 1973, pp. 95-119.

Part 3
Strategy Formulation

Chapter 7

Identifying Strategic Alternatives

"Organizations which survive and prosper . . . seem to be able to anticipate important trends and to get into position to exploit new opportunities and avoid potential risks. The company and its environment advance in harmony."

—Richard A. Bobbe and Robert H. Schaffer, *Mastering Change: Breakthrough Projects and Beyond*[1]

"The key to growth—even survival—is to stake out a position that is less vulnerable to attack from head-to-head opponents, whether established or new, and less vulnerable to erosion from the direction of buyers, suppliers, and substitute goods. Establishing such a position can take many forms. . . ."

—Michael E. Porter, *Harvard Business Review*[2]

"Strategic planning is . . . positioning an organization so that it can prosper in the future . . . . First, it is about decision making. As Drucker has said, it does not deal with future decisions, but with the futurity of present decisions. Next, there are long-range connotations. Third, strategic planning deals with important topics. Next, it has to do with the inevitable obsolescence of existing products or processes and the provision for new ones to take their places. Finally, it deals with choices related to the organization itself as opposed to personal choices."

—Clark Holloway and William King, *Long Range Planning*[3]

"[G]enerating alternatives is . . . complicated because it takes considerable time and effort to develop options; difficult because it requires new insights and a willingness to look at the problem from a variety of angles instead of from the same perspective; and frightening because it may require admitting that your past and current strategy won't work in the future . . . or that a new management is necessary."

—William E. Rothschild, *Strategic Alternatives: Selection, Development, and Implementation*[4]

Now that management has diagnosed the hospital's situation in light of various internal or external happenings that are likely to affect the functioning of the institution or its future interests, it is now ready to think strategically. Thinking strategically at this point simply means identifying and analyzing the significant issues that signal the need for a change in direction and developing alternative responses to them. A *strategic issue* is any concern, problem, or opportunity that promises to have a significant bearing on the future direction of an institution. Norman McMillan put his finger on the importance of issues in carrying out a hospital strategic management effort by stating that issues are more than problems—they are what keep causing problems, if not fixed. He advises management to "think of an issue as a problem *generator:* resolve it or fix it, and you get rid of a bunch of problems."[5]

Identification

The following questions are designed to pinpoint key issues to which management can respond in an orderly fashion and over which it can reasonably expect to exercise some influence. They enable management to *develop a list of issues, group these issues, pass them through a strategic screen, and select three or four to focus on when developing future strategies and plans.*

- What issues have surfaced as a result of monitoring the external environment and assessing internal strengths and weaknesses?
- Can the issues be grouped into families of fundamental concerns?
- Do all the identified issues have strategic implications to the hospital? Will resolving them significantly affect the long-range direction of the institution?
- Which issues should be confronted at this time? Which ones can be safely postponed?

The number of issues that can be successfully resolved usually is relatively small. In fact, a common failing of many managers is that they attempt to solve all the issues at the same time or else they squander time on matters from which they can generate only marginal returns.

Don't Use a Shotgun Approach to Strategic Management

"Businesses should also be prudent not to take a shotgun approach to strategic management by attempting to concurrently pursue too many strategic options. This approach inevitably creates inequities and inconsistencies in the allocation of resources."
—Allen M. Yurko, *Harvard Business Review*[6]

Timing can be crucial, both in the sense of identifying and tracking issues and of knowing when to tackle them. Emerging issues can signal either impending opportunities or threats. The trick is, of course, to foster alertness in management, to identify and track early, weak signals, and to respond quickly to these signals so that the institution is rarely surprised by or unprepared for new developments. Some issues are so urgent—perhaps even threatening the very survival of the institution—that they must be addressed immediately and forcefully. However, other issues do not necessarily require immediate resolution. Although important, some issues can be considered in subsequent planning efforts. Others can be postponed indefinitely and resurrected only if and when the situation demands action. Again, such decisions are as much matters of good management sense as of timing.

Having focused the hospital's efforts to a few key issues that have strategic implication and that seem to be manageable, the next step is to identify various alternatives to deal with them. It is from these alternatives that future strategy will be determined. Where do strategic alternatives originate? William F. Glueck states that as a starting point, management should consider options consisting of opportunities that it knows about has identified as promising, that it believes will work, or that are not major breaks with past practice (unless the situation is so desperate that radical measures are required).[7] As in the case of issue identification, it is not practical and probably is impossible to consider all alternatives. And yet, a foolhardy approach would be to accept the first option that comes to mind. Generating several reasonable alternatives encourages an orderly evaluation of strengths, weaknesses, feasibility, practicality, acceptability, and tradeoffs of each, resulting in what is often the best choice under the circumstances. The following questions are useful in identifying alternatives:

- What are some possible responses to the key issues in terms of things that management can control?
- Can the specific alternatives be grouped into more general or broader categories that represent significant possible strategic directions?
- What risks are attached to each alternative?
- What criteria should be used in evaluating the alternatives?
- Which alternative represents the best balance between its ability to meet the criteria for evaluation and the risks associated with it?

When identifying strategic alternatives, the concept that strategy has its roots in pure rivalry must be recognized. When two identical armies or corporations oppose each other, the outcome is indeterminate because a condition of symmetry prevails. Only when certain asymmetries or advantages exist is it possible to determine the winner. As Richard P. Rumelt observes, "The winning strategy (as opposed to tactic) is always the same—play only those games in which you have an advantage. Somewhat less mechanistically, one wins games by exploiting asymmetries that make a difference. . . .[Indeed], *a strategy that does not either create or exploit an asymmetry constituting an advantage must be rejected.*"[8]

Creating Strategic Alternatives

What *might we do* in terms of environmental and local market opportunities?

What *can we do* in terms of organizational competence, resources, and culture?

What do *we want to do* in terms of the hospital's mission and the personal values and aspirations of its management, trustees, and medical staff?

What *should we do* in terms of acknowledged obligations to the hospital's community, its patients, and its various stakeholders?

—Adapted from Kenneth R. Andrews, *The Concept of Corporate Strategy*[9]

A wide range of tools for evaluating strategic alternatives is available.[10] Most managers are familiar with the major tools because they employ them in other decision-making situations: when evaluating policy, performance, budgets, plans, and the acquisition of new technology. In addition to determining the advantages of a strategic alternative, several other considerations can be evaluated:[11]

- Consistency of the alternative to the institution's overall mission and goals
- The quality of the supporting processes and analyses used in identifying the alternative
- Reasonableness of the environmental assumptions on which the alternative rests
- Its substantive content
- Its compatibility with the personal values of management and the organization's basic culture.
- The organization's ability to mobilize the necessary resources and its competency to carry out the alternative effectively and efficiently

Two crucial questions must be asked to properly evaluate an alternative: *Will the alternative work? Will it produce the desired results?*

The Basic Question in Evaluating a Strategy or Strategic Alternative

"Suppose that an analyst is presented with a reasonably comprehensive description of an organization, its environment, and a proposed strategy. What criteria can and should be used in evaluating the strategy? There may be many features of the proposed strategy that are attractive, insightful, and potentially effective. It takes, however, only one major flaw to invalidate the strategy. Thus, it is helpful to cast the evaluation problems in terms of the negative logic of hypothesis testing: on what grounds may a proposed strategy be 'refuted' or rejected?"

—Richard P. Rumelt, *Strategic Management: A New View of Business Policy and Planning*[12]

As conditions change in society or in a market, a hospital may require changes in the only area over which its management has any control, that is, its performance (what it does and how it does it). In fact, *if management does not ensure a continuing alignment (fit) of the hospital with its environment by changing its performance (its overall direction and the nature and quality of its operations), its legitimacy (its reason for existence) may become questionable.*[13] In some instances, this can spell disaster for an institution. The following equation is a convenient starting point not only for reviewing, but also for generating strategic alternatives:

Society (outside) conditions + hospital performance = legitimacy

How a hospital responds to change is as much a reflection of its management style as it is a matter of its ability to perceive the need for change. Some institutions prefer *active or offensive* strategies. They anticipate change and prepare for it. Other institutions are content to adopt *passive or defensive* strategies. They simply react after the fact or follow the leaders. Either type of institution can, of course, select active strategies in one set of circumstances and defensive strategies in a different set of circumstances.[14]

Risk Assessment

Peter F. Drucker, noted management consultant and author, suggests considering the following questions when reviewing challenges and opportunities and appropriate responses:

"Is it a risk that we must accept, a risk that is inherent in the nature of the business?

"Is it a risk that we can afford to take?

"Is it a risk that we cannot afford to take?

"Is it a risk that we cannot afford *not* to take?"

—Peter F. Drucker, *Managing for Results*[15]

Hospitals are learning from industry that many alternatives are open to them in coping with change. In a recent compendium on hospital strategic options, Mara Minerva Melum charges hospital leaders to find opportunities in the challenges and constraints that influence hospitals everywhere. These opportunities range from relatively modest changes in services to fundamental changes in institutional mission to corporate restructuring (see figure 11, Range of Strategic Choice: Hospital Strategy). Some merely entail additions to traditional activities; others involve new and unusual options. The particular situation determines whether these opportunities signify growth, shrinkage, or little change.[16]

Major Strategic Alternatives

Understanding the major strategic alternatives or opportunities that many hospitals are considering is an essential step in making subsequent choices among alternative strategic options and in formulating new strategies. These strategies can be grouped as follows:[17]

Closure and survival strategies. The overriding goal of any organization is to survive. Of course, survival is hardly a justifiable end in itself. Its only significance is in permitting the organization to pursue its principal purpose. Survival is simply a necessary condition for getting on with the job.[18] When conditions change drastically—when an institution and its environment no longer fit, when an institution fails to perform in an efficient or effective manner, or when the competition makes it impractical for the institution to hang on—a hospital may reach the point where its only option is to cease operation. Symond R. Gottlieb, who has given considerable thought to this subject over a long period, observed that "Mere existence of a hospital does not extend the right to mean that it must continue to exist or to expand."[19] Again, the issue is legitimacy, that is, maintaining a responsive alignment of the organization's performance and its external conditions.

The history of U.S. hospitals abounds with hospitals, dispensaries, and other health care institutions that were established for a specific, often limited, purpose and that eventually shut their doors or merged with other institutions because the original conditions that spurred their establishment no longer pertained. Tuberculosis hospitals are a familiar example. Changing times, new values, changes in medical practice, changing public expectations, and development of other resources and capabilities tolled the death knell for many such institutions. Their limited purposes became outdated or irrelevant, particularly when other institutions and new arrangements for financing and delivering hospital care led to incorporating these special purposes into broader missions. In short, these institutions lost their legitimacy.[20]

Although the situation is now different in some ways, it has not really changed: outside forces and internal liabilities can still threaten institutional survival.[21] Hospitals with rigid service goals, limited commitments, inadequate financing, socially irrelevant programs, obsolete facilities, deteriorating markets, or diminishing ability to attract physicians, employees, or patients continue to be vulnerable. The inability to keep abreast of competition by offering a suitable array of high-quality services at a reasonable price or to carve an appropriate niche in a local market are emerging as new threats to institutional well being and survival. Strong signals already indicate that, through survival of the fittest, competition may emerge as the method of controlling the supply of hospital beds.

Robert M. Sigmond has proposed what he terms the *Basic Closure Rule.* This rule states that "A hospital that has the four basic commitments will not—as a matter of fact, *cannot*—close. The four basic commitments are a committed governing board, a committed medical staff, a commitment to the community, and a commitment to a decent institutional standard for ethical conduct and relationships. With these four commitments, a hospital is totally immune to closure. These four commitments do not include such things as cash flow, bottom lines, dollars, or capital funds. They do not even mention anything about good management. All these things are important, but they do not guarantee a hospital against closure."[22] There is enough food for thought in this statement to make further comment on survival strategies unnecessary.

The Art of the Small Win

Research findings on organizational effectiveness show that large organizations have learned that most change occurs bit by bit and major change typically emerges over a long period. Also keep in mind the conclusion that "policy making is typically a never ending process of successive steps in which continual nibbling is a substitute for a good bite."[23] Here is some advice on how to succeed at the art of the small win.

"Focus attention on one or at most two major new items. Solve the problems one-by-one.

"Allow the bad to be displaced by the good instead of trying to legislate it out of existence.

"Frequent, consistent, and positive reinforcement is a great shaper of expectations and a strong inducer of change. Make frequent rewards for small completed actions.

"Add new solutions rather than tackle old problems.

"Be on the lookout for opportunities to reinforce activities that are congruent with the organization's overall or eventual purpose. The forward thinking executive scours his in-basket for solutions, bits of completed action to be singled out as exemplars of some larger theme. Support of complete actions typically generates further actions consistent with the rewarded behavior."

—Thomas J. Peters,
Organizational Dynamics[24]

Turnaround strategies. The turnaround or revival of a dying institution is an offshoot of the survival strategy. It usually results from a determined effort to redress the alignment of the organization with its environment by obtaining new financing, making major changes in mission, restructuring, or reversing past policies. Outside help may be required, albeit not always successful, to rejuvenate a dying corporation or hospital. Little hope exists for such an organization, however, if its leaders are unable to adopt new strategies that encompass more than mere survival. In the health care field, *conversion* to other related uses is not an uncommon turnaround strategy.

Retrenchment strategies. Knowing when to abandon a service or to cut back on existing activities is often more important than knowing when to grow or diversify. Planned abandonment of programs and services that no longer fit the purposes of the institution, for which community need is lacking, or that are better provided by other local institutions is a major strategic alternative too often overlooked. Peter Drucker has some sound advice on this subject: "An essential step is deciding what our business is, what it will be, and what it should be, therefore, systematic analysis of all existing prod-

Range of Strategic Choice: Hospital Strategy

Strategic Choice	Range of Choice → A	B	C	D	E	F	G	H	Current/ Future
1. Institutional values	Don't rock the boat	Roll with the punches	Plan ahead	Dream ahead					
2. Reaction to change	Reject	Adapt	Anticipate	Seek					
3. Basic growth strategy	Exit gracefully	Hold position	Increase market share	Grow selectively (specialize)	Diversify away from traditional markets	Pursue vertical integration	Conversion	Closure	
4. Strategic thrust	Driven by outside sanctions and incentives	Driven by capabilities and resources	Driven by results, e.g., financial, quality	Driven by services offered	Driven by markets served	Same as markets served			
5. Community and services	Selected services to selected populations	Selected services to entire service area	Comprehensive services to selected populations	Comprehensive services to entire service area	Combination of these				
6. Role in multi-institutional arrangement	Go it alone	Build on existing affiliations	Become part of a multi-institutional system	Link hospital, physicians, and insurance, e.g., HMO	Become a system builder				
7. Key strategic resources	Medical staff	Nursing and allied health personnel	Management	Financial	Physical plant	Goodwill (community support)	Political clout		
8. Geographic target	Local community	Service area	Beyond traditional service area	Interstate	International				

Issue								
9. Target in levels of health care	Prevention and promotion	Primary and ambulatory care	Secondary inpatient care	Tertiary inpatient care	Long-term care	Rehabilitative care	Terminally ill care	Home health services
10. Quality of care basis	Adequacy of facilities and equipment	Quality of nursing care and performance	Presence and quality of house staff	Quality of medical staff and physician performance	Quality of allied health and supervisory staff	Quality of organizational coordinator and management	Overall patient care and patient reaction	Comparative overall care
11. Leadership in medical technology	No follow	Slow follow	Quick follow	Innovative leadership				
12. Financial strategy	Accept reimbursement as limit	Maximize reimbursement	Seek new sources of revenue					
13. Management of external affairs	Independent response, voluntary public relations	Cooperation	Cooptation	Coalition forming and joining	Alter the environment			
14. Graduate medical education	No residency	Limited number of residencies	Broad array of residencies	Limited affiliation with medical school	Major affiliation with medical school			
15. Nursing education	None	Clinical affiliation	Diploma nursing school	Baccalaureate or associate degree program	LPN school			
16. Research	None	Limited to clinical research	Combined clinical and basic research	Basic research	Cooperate with university or research institute			

Figure 11. Shown above are some of the issues facing a hospital and the range of possible choices for dealing with each issue. The choices selected then form the hospital's strategy.

ucts, processes, markets, and uses, and distribution channels. Are they still viable? And are they likely to remain viable? Do they still give value to the customer? And are they likely to do so tomorrow? Do they still fit the realities of population and markets, of technology and economy? And if not, how can we best abandon them—or at least stop pouring in further resources and efforts?''[25] Product portfolio analysis, described later in this chapter, is a helpful tool in making such decisions.

Retrenchment is almost always an unpopular alternative. To some, it indicates a cautious conservativism that is not conducive to vitality and growth. The above observations should convince these persons otherwise. Retrenchment and planned abandonment are simply two of the many alternatives for ensuring a responsive alignment of an organization and its changing environment. Nor is it a sign of failure or a pessimistic portent.

Growth strategies. As with many other industries, hospitals have traditionally followed one or more growth strategies. Many have successfully done so as outgrowths of a conscious, active strategy, at times in advance of a demonstrated need. In fact, as the well-known Roemer's Law postulates, under conditions of widespread prepayment, the existing supply of hospital beds determines their use and this, in turn, stimulates adding more beds.[26] Although circumstances have changed dramatically in recent years because of regulatory and reimbursement controls, many hospitals continue to explore opportunities for growth and expansion on the assumption that the market for their services either needs more beds or will support them in any event.

Several growth alternatives have been described in corporate strategy literature.[27] The most frequent, *incremental growth,* occurs when a firm regards itself as successful and from time to time perceives a need for growth. Hospitals have historically adopted this alternative. Many have prepared long-range master plans for future development of facilities and services, which assume the continuous availability of resources, an increasing market, and a sustained, growing demand for services. When conditions are ripe, such as when occupancy pressures reach an intolerable level or the medical staff demands it, a decision may be made by the hospital's governing board to add beds by constructing new facilities or renovating existing space. This decision relieves the pressure or satisfies staff demands until the process is repeated. Indeed, this ad-hoc pattern has dominated most hospital planning ventures in the past.

In itself, incremental growth is not necessarily bad or undesirable. Only when the growth is haphazard or when the decision to do so is impetuous, with little regard for long-term consequences or community needs, is the practice foolhardly and, perhaps, counterproductive. In addition, growth need not be limited to facilities; it may embrace products and services and extend to vertical integration and other organizational arrangements.

Despite the warnings by many knowledgeable persons in the health care field that future hospital growth is limited and that retrenchment and exploration of new roles are the most promising directions for the future, little evidence exists to indicate that hospitals are turning away from their traditional preoccupations with new construction, acquisition of new technology, and adding services. One need only attend local or state hearings on certificate-of-need and section 1122 of the Social Security Act to realize how much emphasis is still being placed on growth (mainly construction) strategies by hospitals, nursing homes, and other health care organizations in many parts of the United States.

Development strategies. Development is not a synonym for growth, although many managers and planners are prone to use the two terms interchangeably. Growth involves an *increase in size or number;* development denotes an *increase in capacity or potential.* ''Growth can take place with or without development, and development can take place with or without growth.''[28] When a hospital searches for better ways to satisfy its own desires and the expectations of its stakeholders, to do more with less or with the same resources, to enhance its management capabilities, or in some other way to strengthen its competencies, it is obviously pursuing a different strategy (both in kind and direction) than when, for example, it adds beds, inaugurates a new service, or constructs an annex.

What's the Big Rush?

''Be cautious of technological temptations! Learn to differentiate between being a pioneer and being an innovator. The definition of a pioneer, a friend of mine said, 'is to get the arrow in the back.' Someone will always be the pioneer. But there is no reason for the same institution to always be the pioneer. Some pioneers will be heavily subsidized by the sponsors of what they're pioneer-

> ing with, and that's as it should be. Wait until the data come in; wait until you see the cost effectiveness; wait until there's a hard data base upon which to make decisions. The quality of health care in this country is so good today that I cannot understand why people feel compelled to make major technological innovations today, rather than wait 12 or 24 months. What is the downside risk? It's very small. Wait until you have the information you need to make a decision. . . . Don't [just] pick up the dice and roll them across the table and say, "Well, it's only a million dollars. If it works out, great; if it doesn't, at least we have the best piece of equipment."
>
> —Peter Carpenter, speech[29]

Development strategies are particularly appropriate when resources are scarce, such as in many parts of the Third World, or when competition for limited resources is strong, such as in communities where hospitals are fiercely competing for funds, physicians, nurses, and patients. Resource limitations do not necessarily limit development; in many instances, a lack of resources spurs development. Moreover, development strategies often lead to consideration of diversification, collaborative arrangements, market niche strategies, recruitment, and other alternatives.

Opportunistic strategies. Many hospitals seem not to have formally expressed strategies. They respond to opportunities as they arise and make little or no effort to track new developments. They are simply freewheeling opportunists. This method can be a valid strategic approach in some instances, particularly for small hospitals with modest managerial capabilities and limited resources. With experience, however, these institutions may wish to turn to other more aggressive strategic alternatives.

Collaborative arrangements. Hospitals are turning to a variety of collaborative arrangements in their efforts to contain costs, increase services, counter external threats, and capitalize on new opportunities. Mergers, affiliations, consortiums, shared services, multihospital systems, federations, contract management, lease arrangements, hospital chains and other joint ownership ventures, and "unbundled" management assistance are familiar strategies. These arrangements arise from a recognition that hospitals provide a variety of services, many of which are produced in such low volume that their costs are too high or are so infrequently used that the income to support them is often inadequate. And small hospitals simply aren't large enough economically to do most of the things they attempt to do.

Much has been written about collaborative arrangements in the hospital field.[30] Some words on *multi-institutional arrangements* do, however, seem to be in order. Not only are many being developed nationwide, but they also involve an increasing array of health care programs and facilities: community hospitals, nursing homes, mental hospitals, home health care services, prepaid medical plans, satellite operations, and other health care services. A recent journal reported that 176 hospital systems owned, leased, and managed 29 percent of the total 5,842 nonfederal, short-term general community hospitals in the United States and 30 percent of the 984,000 community hospital beds. This report also optimistically forecasted that both the number of hospitals and beds in these multi-institutional arrangements will continue to grow.[31]

These arrangements involve not-for-profit organizations, including religious entities; investor-owned companies; and public hospitals (usually local government-owned). Health Central, Inc., Intermountain Health Care, Fairview Community Hospitals, Lutheran Hospitals and Homes Society, the four Adventist health systems, and the Sisters of Mercy Health Corporation are examples of large not-for-profit groups that own, lease, and manage substantial numbers of institutions and beds. Hospital Corporation of America and American Medical International are investor-owned chains that are among the largest in terms of beds and investment.

These multi-institutional systems vary considerably in programs and relationships. They entail almost any arrangement or practice, including establishing or constructing new hospitals, purchasing or leasing existing facilities, contract managing, sharing services, purchasing in groups, consulting assistance, and providing various other centralized planning, development, consultative, and management support activities. Some are designed to provide the benefits of consolidation while retaining local autonomy and identity for their various units.[32]

Many hospitals are exploring these and other collaborative ventures as worthwhile options for coping with the future. But joining a multi-unit system is rarely an easy decision for an institution. Such ventures almost always entail long-range commitment of resources and demand a broader outlook than hospital leaders may be accustomed to take. In addition, despite their increasing popularity, collaborative strategies may not be an appropriate or workable alternative in a hospital's particular situation. However, some experts contend that collaborative strategies are always viable possibilities that should be rejected only for substantial reasons.

Market strategies. Most hospitals have followed a nonmarketing or even an antimarketing approach in attending to their customers. "Their basic philosophy has been that they should provide the best possible services as they see them, and they hope enough people will make use of those services to make their efforts worthwhile. In other words, the organization decides what it wants to do, and the public is supposed to be willing to have it done to them.[33]

Of course, all hospitals do some marketing, but until recently, they have not always been willing to admit it.

Marketing concepts and applications can be used by hospitals in developing strategic alternatives. Two principal market strategies are possible: dominate a particular segment of the market by providing something unique or different—the *market niche* alternative—or take an almost opposite approach and strive to increase the market served—the *market share* alternative. The latter strategy is for leaders, "not for the timid or followers, and successful pursuit of this strategy appears limited to a few companies in any industry. Others are relegated to market niche approaches or marginal participation in the mainstream."[34]

Narrowing the market by focusing on a single or limited product can be a risky, but sometimes highly successful strategy. With this approach, an institution opts to concentrate on an activity that it does best, such as family medicine or a specialty service such as rehabilitation. The continuing success of a handful of special hospitals such as Massachusetts Eye and Ear Infirmary in Boston, Wills Eye Hospital in Philadelphia, and Oklahoma Children's Memorial Hospital in Oklahoma City is evidence that *if the proper focus is chosen and local market conditions are supportive,* a hospital can restrict its role to a specialty or to a limited constituency. However, as already noted, many hospitals that have pursued this strategy in the past were unable to survive.

Product portfolio or service mix strategies. Strategies based on product portfolio analysis are popular, and various matrixes and tools have been designed to enable organizations to carry them out (see figure 12, Portfolio Analysis). Indeed, some consultants seem almost to equate strategic thinking with portfolio or service mix analysis. Despite some tendency to overapply the technique, portfolio analysis is a useful tool for alerting management to the important interrelationships that exist among a hospital's service mix and market growth opportunities. The technique assists management in breaking a habit of rewarding profitable activities with bigger budgets while starving less attractive activities with lean budgets. Like any other business, a hospital must produce services and products that generate cash, because cash is needed to pay its bills and to keep its doors open. Unlike many other businesses, hospitals also need cash to finance low-market (usually specialized) activities, such as burn centers, maternity units, and other money losers that are essential to its community. The challenge for hospitals exists in balancing the product mix with other market and community considerations.[35]

Diversification. Diversification strategies are increasingly part of the hospital scene. Hospitals are redefining their historic role as providers of acute care inpatient services. Many are considering other service options, and some are even making fundamental changes in the scope and types of services they provide or expect to provide in the future. Adding new products and services, indeed, even adding totally unrelated products through acquisition of other firms, is a common business strategy. Scarcely a day passes without a press announcement that a company has added a new product line or acquired or merged another firm, thus adding significant new business interests or products.

A diverse and expanding product line is usually regarded as an asset, with two caveats: a firm should concentrate only on products for which demand is strong and growing and should consider only new products or services that it already knows how to manage or for which it can quickly develop the capabilities to do so.

It is easy to be tempted into believing that diversification is a panacea to market problems. In their efforts to copy industry, hospitals are apt to overlook that some of the world's most successful businesses have only one product line, one major market, and one central technology. Peter Drucker warns that diversification may only add to an organization's troubles and that the more complex the business, the more things can go wrong and the more difficult it is to take corrective action. He recommends two questions as a starting point for evaluating a diversification strategy: "What is the *least*

Portfolio Analysis

Portfolio analysis, particularly the Boston Consulting Group's four-box matrix, is a familiar tool used by multiproduct firms to channel resources into their most productive units. The figure below is used in many strategic planning or marketing texts and workshop sessions.

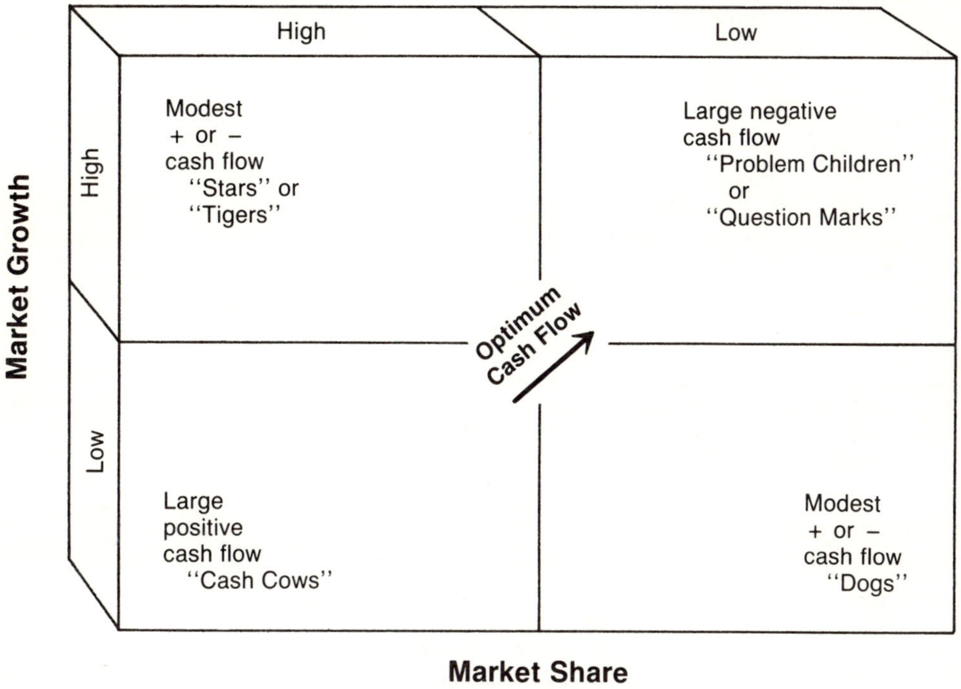

Products or services to the left of the Market Share dividing line (the Stars and Cash Cows) have strong cash flows from operations, and those to the right have weaker or negative cash flows. Products or services below the market growth dividing line require little investment to maintain their market share, and those above the line need substantial cash investments to keep abreast of market growth. Good management aims to keep enough Cash Cows to feed the Problem Children and to encourage the Problem Children to become Stars rather than Dogs.[36]

Although many hospitals provide a diverse array of discrete products and services, portfolio analysis is not as useful for them as it is for other business enterprises. As designed, the tool makes no provision for examining an institution's social role and contributions, important considerations that must be taken into account in analyzing a hospital's growth-share of a given market. Some poly-matrix constructs devised by McKinsey & Company and others, however, do supply a somewhat broader product analysis perspective. All are useful tools for encouraging market-oriented strategic thinking.

Figure 12. A portfolio analysis matrix alerts management to the interrelationships that exist among a hospital's service mix and market growth opportunities.

diversification this business needs to accomplish its mission, obtain its objectives, and continue to be viable and prosperous? What is the *most* diversification we can manage, the most complexity this business can bear?''[37]

The following services and arrangements represent most, but certainly not all, of the present diversification possibilities available to hospitals:

- Hospices
- Family planning services
- Long-term care
- Swing-bed arrangements
- Ambulatory care
- Satellite or outreach clinics
- Emergicenters
- Medical office buildings
- Home health services
- Mental health programs
- Crisis intervention
- Health hazard appraisal
- Contract management for other health care institutions
- Industrial health programs
- Medical surveillance for industry
- Stress management
- Occupational and environmental health services
- Rehabilitation services
- Health screening
- Nutrition and obesity programs
- Wellness programs, health promotion, and aerobics
- Sports medicine
- Holistic health programs
- Health education
- Alternative healing and therapy activities
- Medical care cooperatives
- Health maintenance organizations
- Family-centered health services
- Alcoholism programs (inpatient and outpatient)
- Other substance abuse programs

In addition to the above health-related activities, numerous unrelated opportunities exist, such as parking garages, hotel or motel accommodations for visitors and guests, congregate housing, consultative services, catered condominiums, and other income-producing ventures. In fact, a multihospital system recently acquired a law school and plans to channel income from this operation into health care-related activities. Although some of these ventures may seem inappropriate in light of traditional hospital commitments, they represent feasible strategic growth or diversification options.

Diversification is often pursued in the quest for growth. It also is a means of moving out of declining traditional activities that are becoming less profitable and of substituting new products or services with greater growth potential or income-producing expectations.

Recruitment strategies. Hospitals face the persistent problem of attracting and retaining a core of qualified physicians and other practitioners of the healing arts who are not only committed to the goals of the institution, but also are willing to refer patients in sufficient numbers to support the institution's programs and services. Hospitals in small communities or in sparsely settled areas with limited health manpower resources are particularly susceptible to the problem of physician shortages. In addition, many large and small hospitals are encountering increasing difficulties in meeting nursing staff requirements.

As Jeff C. Goldsmith has wisely observed, ''Since the key to hospital use is an active, committed medical staff, recruiting and retaining physicians are the most important marketing issues facing hospital managers."[38] In addition, many new diversification options, such as the establishment of emergicenters, satellite clinics, industrial health programs, and health maintenance organizations (HMOs), require cadres of physicians and paraprofessionals who are willing to participate in these programs. New strategies are often needed to attract them to these less conventional ventures.

Recruitment problems can limit a hospital's strategic options and can lead to retrenchment strategies or even to closure. Therefore, recruitment issues often dominate the strategic planning efforts of many hospitals.

Financial strategies. Although finances permeate virtually every strategic alternative, some financial strategies merit special and distinct consideration. They focus on the basic ways that hospitals generate funds for capital expenditures and for current operations. Because most hospitals have been unable to build up capital reserves, they have, as a matter of tradition, been forced to turn to outside sources including the federal government, for funds to underwrite new construction, finance new ventures, or purchase major items of equipment. Only a generation ago a leading monograph on the United States hospital reported that "practically all the hospital capital in this country has come through the medium of voluntary contributions or by taxation."[39] The thought of turning to the commercial bond market or to pursuing the tax-exempt bond route for raising venture capital was until recently anathema to most voluntary hospital authorities. For example, a great teacher of an entire past generation of hospital administrators, Malcolm T. MacEachern, advised against the use of bonds as a means of finance. "There are two good reasons for emphasizing this point. The first is that in most instances the hospital cannot earn sufficient [funds] to meet any indebtedness beyond cost of operation; and the second, that if it is organized as not-for-profit it is not justified in using any surplus which may accrue from operation for retiring or paying interest on capital indebtedness."[40] This advice seems strange today, but it does emphasize the point that *changing times generate new strategies to address old issues.*

Financial Strategies for Hospitals

"If the hospital doesn't have a strong financial base, why not consider formal economic consolidations with other organizations to achieve a stronger capital position? Such arrangements don't necessarily require the existing board to lose control or change policy. . . .

"Additionally, corporate reorganizations, possibly in conjunction with capital restructuring or the formation of limited partnership arrangements, should be considered as a means of sheltering certain assets. This may not be appropriate in every situation; restructuring can result in more harm than good if implemented only because it's the newest catchword. . . .

"Optimum strategies exist even in an adverse environment. Therefore, trustees should actively direct the development of a comprehensive plan to ensure the future viability of their institution."
—Frank J. Grimmelmann,
Trustee[41]

George A. Steiner states that "There are three ways to go broke running a business. One is to spend too much, another is to spend too little, and the third is to invest in the wrong thing."[42] Thus, a good strategy involves seeking ways to avert these possibilities. Costs of hospital operation should be held to the lowest possible level consistent with the institution's goals and accepted standards; however, to be really effective, cost containment efforts must reflect long-term continuing commitments to greater efficiency and higher productivity that, in turn, are based on well-designed strategies. Moreover, these strategies must be recognized as distinct from budgets that deal mainly with short-term (usually annual) operating targets.

In short, because all aspects of a hospital's operations are in one way or another affected by its finances and by the general state of the economy, hospitals must always be alert to new strategic options that will enable them to generate and employ the required funds to carry out their mission and long-term goals.

Competitive strategies. A competitive strategy is the means an organization uses to find a position in its industry or market to best defend itself against the five competitive forces described in chapter 4 or influence these forces to its advantage. An essential starting point in developing such a strategy is an analysis of corporate strengths and weaknesses (see chapter 6), particularly those aspects of the organization's behavior that disclose its attitude toward substitute or new services and its capacity to position itself in relation to new entrants and other local competitive forces. Actually, as Michael E. Porter observes, "Strategy can be viewed as building defenses against the competitive forces or as finding positions in the industry where the forces are weakest."[43] However, *this requires insights into the organization's capabilities and the causes of outside competitive forces so that the organization can decide when and where to confront the competition or how to avoid it.*

Competition: A Word Searching for Respectability in the Health Care Field

"Recently, the word *competition* has become a rallying cry throughout the health care system, with some groups insisting that widespread economic competition in health care could reduce costs, eliminate irrational disincentives, and restructure the provision of health care. Opponents of the idea say that a competitive environment would cripple the system and deny access to many patients. The very mention of competition leads to debates about regulation, deregulation, pluralism, free enterprise, and other economic issues.

"Perhaps the first thing that should be noted is the fact that the word *competition* is being used as a rubric to identify a wide range of theories and proposals designed to alter current health care practice. Virtually none of these proposals involves turning the provision of health care into a total, free-market, price-controlled process; few products or services are bought and sold with no restrictions whatever, and long-standing social policy ensures that health care would never be left to an uncontrolled economic environment. What health care experts mean when they say 'competition' is the introduction of certain specific mechanisms into the system to encourage people and institutions to behave differently from the way they have traditionally behaved. As Victor Fuchs, Ph.D., says, the ideas that are at issue are 'market mechanisms and market forces,' not traditional competition. Health economist C. Rufus Rorem, Ph.D., describes the unstated public policy as 'Competition may be the life of trade, but health care is not private property to be bought and sold in a competitive market.' "

—Emily Friedman,
Hospitals[44]

An organization can devise an offensive strategy that enables it to cope directly with competitive forces or it can stake out a position that makes it less vulnerable to these forces. Specifically, an organization can fight for its market share by improving its services, its image, or its products, or by lowering its prices without sacrificing quality. It can solidify its relationships with favored customers, such as relieving physicians of various medical record and administrative chores or negotiating price inducements with a large-scale, third-party purchaser. It can add substitute or new services in an attempt to expand its market. It can raise various barriers to entry, thereby discouraging new competition. For example, many hospitals have supported tight certificate-of-need regulatory controls in their states; and some nursing home associations, with the encouragement and support of their members, have adopted a hard-line attitude to new entrants by contesting proposals for additional or new facilities at state and local certificate-of-need hearings. In addition, an organization can even take actions that drive out a weak competitor, perhaps by establishing a satellite facility or outreach program that would threaten or in other ways harm its competitors, such as stealing a prominent specialist or heavy admitter from a neighboring institution.[45] Obviously, many value and ethical considerations affect such decisions (see chapter 8).

Brinkmanship Strategies

The heart of a company's business strategy or, for that matter, a diplomatic or military strategy is to promote attitudes on the part of its competitors that will frighten them into restraining themselves or cause them to act in a fashion that management considers advantageous. There are five rules for accomplishing this:

1. Determine as accurately as possible just what your competitor has at stake in his contact with you. The issue is not what you stand to gain or lose, but what he stands to gain or lose that limits his ability to compromise with you
2. The less the competition knows about what you intend to do and the risks involved,

the less his advantage. Without such a reference point, he does not even know whether you are being unreasonable in your contact with him.

3. Knowing the character, attitudes, motives, and habitual behavior of your competitors is absolutely essential if you are seeking a negotiating advantage.
4. If you make your demands more arbitrary your competitor position will improve—provided you do not elicit an emotional response.
5. On the other hand, the less arbitrary you seem to be, the more arbitrary you can in fact be.

These rules constitute "the art of business brinkmanship." They are simply guidelines for achieving a strategic victory in your competitors' minds. Once achieved, it can be converted into a competitive victory in terms of sales volume, costs, profits, and market position.

—Adapted, with permission,
from Bruce B. Henderson,
Henderson on Corporate Strategy[46]

Defensive strategies. Not all strategies are aggressive or opportunistic. Some are clearly defensive and are usually pursued to protect an organization against the actions of its competitors, to avert emerging threats to its continued well-being, or to survive in a period of limited or diminishing resources. But a defensive strategy is more than simply an option among many options: it is a basic attitude, or a frame of mind that directs management to cut back, redirect, consolidate, or phase out some of its programs and activities.[47]

At the prodding of health planning agencies, local community organizations, and other outside groups, and often accompanied by special grants or government financial assistance, many hospitals initiated programs that unexpectedly overtaxed their resources or that proved unsatisfactory in other ways. For example, in the late 1960s, some hospitals established ambulatory clinics in inner cities with the help of Office of Economic Opportunity funds. When the funds were withdrawn, many of these programs turned into liabilities for the sponsoring hospitals. Similarly, many hospitals also added long-term care units in a laudable attempt to develop into comprehensive health service centers, which was then considered the balanced hospital community, only to discover later that they were unable to finance these ventures because of reimbursement limitations. When measured in terms of organizational vitality and effectiveness, discontinuing such endeavors may have represented the best strategy at the time.

Some organizations also pursue defensive strategies that force competitors to back down or to avoid potential conflict altogether. Michael E. Porter observes that the cornerstone of such a defense is an organization's commitment to "guarantee the likelihood, speed, and vigor of retaliation to offensive moves." In fact, "if a firm appears unbeatable, a battle is unlikely to occur."[48]

Obviously, many hospitals have successfully protected their markets by adopting defensive strategies. They seem to be able to communicate an aura of unbeatability that discourages competition from other providers, either *by deed,* such as through the scope and quality of services offered, their ability to attract outstanding staffs, their access to philanthropic funds, or their superior facilities, or *by word,* such as through skillful public and community relations. They also seem able to convince would-be competitors that certain moves are unwise or unprofitable. Some institutions have turned certificate-of-need hearings to their advantage by seizing these opportunities to denounce proposals for new facilities and services by local competitors as unneeded, too costly, or impossible to staff. In some instances, several local institutions have banded together in class actions to contest the application of a new entrant into their market. These moves are not necessarily successful, as the recent building of the City of Faith in Tulsa, OK, attests.

With the promise of greater competition in health care, institutions may find it necessary to consider defensive strategies designed to overcome weaknesses that make them especially vulnerable to change. Or, they may consider such strategies in order to protect themselves against the encroachment of other institutions competing in the same market for patients, physicians, employees, and funds. However, many may soon discover, that a good offense is often the best defense and to counter the competition will turn to the positive strategies described elsewhere in this chapter.

Corporate restructuring or reorganizing. With some exceptions as a result of variations in auspices, a typical hospital is a single entity based on a familiar, traditional model and exempt from federal and state income taxes. But this model may no longer be completely satisfactory to accommodate new demands and opportunities. Most hospitals' existing corporate structures do not, for example, allow them to maximize third-party reimbursement or to undertake activities unrelated to original corporate purposes without jeopardizing their tax-exempt status.

Rules for Carrying out Corporate Restructuring

Spin off all reimbursable cost centers and low reimbursable centers, at least those that are physically separate.

Do not conduct new noninstitutional health services in hospital corporation.

Provide clear links of authority and control.

Do not create nontaxable events into taxable activities.

Combine taxable activities into a single for-profit corporation to offset taxable losses against taxable income. Run some numbers through proposal to evaluate results.

There is not "only one way to fly."

Proceed slowly: only shift functions, resources, and personnel after an appropriate study of advantages and disadvantages has been made.

Any system, no matter how well organized, needs imaginative leadership and direction.
—Ross E. Stromberg, handout[49]

In searching for new organizational alternatives to cope with change, some hospitals are turning to *holding company arrangements, investor-owned subsidiaries, quasi-independent development foundations, wholly independent foundations,* and various *joint-venture models.*[50] Each option has its advantages and disadvantages. Therefore, careful evaluation is essential in reviewing these alternatives (see Rules for Carrying Out Corporate Restructuring).

Much overlap exists in the preceding strategic alternatives. Indeed, the list has been somewhat contrived for grouping purposes. It is, for example, not easy to draw a line between a product portfolio strategy and diversification. Turnaround and retrenchment strategies are often simply survival or defensive strategies. Market strategies support various recruitment, diversification, and conversion efforts. Financial strategies are interlaced with growth and opportunistic strategies and, indeed, with any other alternative that requires the acquisition or outlay of funds to support the strategy. Thus, it can be expected that a hospital will consider several, often interrelated strategic alternatives and will select one or several of them as it attempts to better position itself for future change. The next chapter explores how these choices are made.

Notes

1. Bobbe, Richard A., and Schaffer, Robert H. *Mastering Change: Breakthrough Projects and Beyond.* AMA Management Bulletin no. 120. New York City: American Management Association, 1968.
2. Porter, Michael E. How competitive forces shape strategy. *Harvard Business Review.* 57:137, Mar.-Apr. 1979.
3. Holloway, Clark, and King, William R. Evaluating alternative approaches to strategic planning. *Long Range Planning.* 12:75, Aug. 1979.
4. Rothschild, William E. *Strategic Alternatives: Selection, Development, and Implementation.* New York City: AMACOM, 1979, pp. vii-viii.
5. McMillan, Norman H. *Planning for Survival: A Handbook for Hospital Trustees.* Chicago: American Hospital Association, 1978. The chapter "Issue-Oriented Planning: Facing the Music" is full of advice on handling the issues that many hospitals face, some of which are often "unspeakable."
6. Yurko, Allen M. In letter. *Harvard Business Review.* 59:180, Jan.-Feb. 1981.
7. Glueck, William F. *Strategic Management and Business Policy.* New York City: McGraw-Hill Book Company, 1980, p. 200.

8. Rumelt, Richard P. *Evaluation of strategy: theory and models.* In: Schendel, Dan E., and Hofer, Charles W., editors. *Strategic Management: A New View of Business Policy and Planning.* Boston: Little, Brown & Company, 1979, pp. 202-03.

9. Andrews, Kenneth R. The Concept of Corporate Strategy. Homewood, IL: Richard D. Irwin, Inc., 1980, p. 26.

10. For more on methods of evaluation, see Steiner, George A., and Miner, John B. *Management Policy and Strategy.* New York City: MacMillan Publishing Co., Inc., 1977; Schendel and Hofer, chapter 4 and accompanying paper by Rumelt, Richard P. and commentary by Kirchoff, Bruce A.; and Glueck, chapter 5.

11. An elaboration and adaptation of a listing in Schendel and Hofer, pp. 190-2.

12. Rumelt, Richard P. Evaluation of strategy: theory and models. In: Schendel, Dan E., and Hofer, Charles W., editors. *Strategic Management: A New View of Business Policy and Planning.* Boston: Little, Brown and Company, 1979, p. 199.

13. Sethi, S. Prahash. A conceptual framework for environmental analysis of social issues and evaluation of business response patterns. *Academy of Management Review.* 4:63, 1979.

14. For more on a basic strategic preference and for a typology of an organization's past strategies on this active/passive dimension, see Glueck, pp. 199-200.

15. Drucker, Peter F. *Managing for Results.* London: Pan Books in association with Heinemann, 1967, pp. 234-5.

16. Minnesota Hospital Association. *The Changing Role of the Hospital: Options for the Future.* Chicago: American Hospital Association, 1980, p. 3. There is much information and advice in this book that is extremely useful in generating strategic options for hospitals as they face what the editor describes as "a turning point fraught with difficult adjustments."

17. The list of major strategic alternatives is derived from McCarthy, Daniel J., and others. *Business Policy and Strategy: Concepts and Readings.* Homewood, IL: Richard D. Irwin, Inc., 1979, pp. 311 ff., with additional alternatives from Glueck, pp. 202 ff.

18. Chamberlain, Neil W. *Enterprise and Environment: The Firm in Time and Place.* New York City: McGraw-Hill, Inc., 1968, p. 45.

19. Gottlieb, S. R. Reducing excess hospital capacity is a tough but necessary job. *Hospitals.* 52:63, Dec. 1, 1978.

20. See, for example, Fifield, James Clark. *American and Canadian Hospitals.* Chicago: Physicians' Record Company, 1937. This early source lists special hospitals in virtually every state and major city in the late 1930s. In addition to the ubiquitous tuberculosis hospital, there were many types of special institutions organized in the late 19th and early 20th centuries to serve emerging medical specialties and prevalent disease groupings: women's hospitals, homeopathic hospitals, isolation hospitals, smallpox hospitals, lying-in hospitals, orthopedic hospitals, maternity hospitals, babies' hospitals, skin and cancer hospitals, hospitals for mental and nervous diseases, convalescent hospitals, hospitals for epileptics, children's hospitals, hospitals for contagious diseases, and hospitals for eye, ear, nose, and throat diseases. Also, early in the 20th century, institutions that owed their origin and support to church groups representing every major denomination and many splinter groups accounted for as much as 40 or more percent of all voluntary hospitals in the United States. In some large, old cities mainly on the East Coast, hospitals were also organized to meet the special needs of various groups who had emigrated to and settled in the area. New York City once had an Italian hospital, a Chinese hospital, a Swedish hospital, and an Austro-Hungarian hospital. Philadelphia had a German hospital, as did several other cities until the hysteria of World War I frightened hospital authorities into changing the names of these institutions to Lankenau Hospital (Philadelphia), Lenox Hill Hospital (New York City), and Research Hospital (Kansas City). Baltimore and Chicago each had a Provident Hospital, with all-black medical staffs, which catered to the needs of local black populations. In addition, dozens of industrial hospitals were established by railroad companies (A.T. & S.F. Hospitals in Topeka, KS, Albuquerque, NM, and Fort Madison, IA; Missouri Pacific Hospital in Little Rock, AR; and Southern Pacific Hospital in Houston), by manufacturers (Stetson Hospital in Philadelphia; General Electric Company Industrial Hospital in Schenectady, NY; and Goodyear Hospital and Dispensary in Akron, OH), and other industries (Kennecott Copper Corporation Hospital in Kennecott, AK, Republic Mining and Manufacturing Company Hospital in Bauxite, AR, and Lumbermen's Hospital in Bend, OR) to provide hospital services to company employees.

21. See Pleines, Karen M., and Williams, Herbert. Planning with the community can prevent hospital closings. *Hospitals.* 52:87, Dec. 1, 1978; and papers on closure and conversion in Minnesota Hospital Association. *The Changing Role of the Hospital: Options for the Future.* Chicago: American Hospital Association, 1980. Also, U.S. Department of Health and Human Services, PHS, HRA, Bureau of Health Facilities. *Hospital Closure: Findings, Conclusions, and Recommendations on Employee Issues and Consideration for Facility Conversion.* Final Report, May 1980. HRP-090247. Available from National Technical Information Service, Springfield, VA 22161.

22. Sigmond, Robert M. An open-minded approach to hospital closure. In: Minnesota Hospital Association. *The Changing Role of the Hospital: Options for the Future.* Chicago: American Hospital Association, 1980, p. 315.

23. Lindblom, Charles E. The science of 'muddling through.' *Public Administration Review.* 19:79, Spring 1959.

24. See Peters, Thomas J. Symbols, patterns, and settings: an optimistic case for getting things done. *Organizational Dynamics.* 7:2, Autumn 1978.

25. Drucker, Peter E. *Management: Tasks-Responsibilities-Practices.* New York City; Harper & Row, Publishers, 1974, p. 94.

26. See Klarman, Herbert E. Planning for facilities. In: Ginzberg, Eli, editor. *Regionalization and Health Policy* (Publication no. HRA 77-623). Washington, DC: HEW, 1977.

27. The subject of growth strategies is treated in Glueck, pp. 201 ff., and by Kefalos, A. G. The case for a sustainable growth strategy. In: Glueck, appended to chapter 5.

28. Ackoff, Russell L. *Creating the Corporate Future.* New York City: John Wiley & Sons, 1981, p. 34.

29. Carpenter, Peter. Speech to the Society for Hospital Planning, San Francisco, May 4, 1981.

30. Recent publications on hospital collaborative arrangements include: Zukerman, Howard S., principal author, and Weeks, Lewis E., editor. *Multi-Institutional Hospital Systems.* Chicago: Hospital Research and Educational Trust, 1979; Cochrane, John D., and Fourkas, Ted, editors. *Hospital Consortia: Are They Just Another Layer of Bureaucracy? Or a Key to Survival?* Sacramento: California Hospital Association, 1979; and Hepner, James O., editor. *Health Planning for Emerging Multihospital Systems.* St. Louis: The C. V. Mosby Company, 1978. Also, for a recent review of the literature, see Brown, Montague. Systems diversify with ventures outside the hospital. *Hospitals.* 55:147, Apr. 1, 1981.

31. Johnson, Donald E. L., and Di Paolo, Vince. Multihospital system survey: $1.7 million Kaiser on top. *Modern Healthcare.* 11:79, Apr. 1981.

32. Platou, Carl, and Rice, James. Multihospital holding companies. *Harvard Business Review.* May-June 1972.

33. MacStravic, Robin E. *Marketing Health Care.* Germantown, MD: Aspen Systems Corporation, 1977, p. x.

34. McCarthy and others, p. 316.

35. Product portfolio planning is reported to be losing some of its past luster and some consultants who have been preaching the concept are now downplaying it. See America's restructured economy. *Business Week.* June 1, 1981, p. 88; Haspeslagh, Phillip. Portfolio planning: uses and limits. *Harvard Business Review.* 60:58, Jan.-Feb. 1982; and Pekar, Peter P. Jr., Portfolio analysis: a planner's dilemma. *Planning Review.* 10:14, July 1982.

36. See Abell, Derek F., and Hammond, John S. *Strategic Market Planning: Problems and Analytical Approaches.* Englewood Cliffs, NJ: Prentice-Hall, Inc., 1979, pp. 176-9, for discussion of this figure in developing portfolio strategies; also see Glueck, pp. 162-4.

37. Drucker, 1974, p. 692.

38. Goldsmith, Jeff C. The health care market: can hospitals survive? *Harvard Business Review.* 52:103, Sept.-Oct. 1980.

39. Corwin, E. H. L. *The American Hospital.* New York City: The Commonwealth Fund, 1946, p. 46. For an update on trends in capital financing for hospitals, see Lightle, Mary Alice. '70s see new approaches to capital financing for hospitals. *Hospitals.* 52:135, June 16, 1978.

40. MacEachern, Malcolm T. *Hospital Organization and Management.* Chicago: Physician's Record Company, 1946, pp. 51-2.

41. Grimmelmann, Frank J. Why hospitals must focus on capital formation. *Trustee.* 34:11, Oct. 1981.

42. Steiner, George A. *Top Management Planning.* New York City: The Macmillan Company, 1969, p. 598.

43. Porter, 1979, p. 137.

44. Friedman, Emily. Does market competition belong in health care? *Hospitals.* 54:47, July, 1980.

45. A summary and adaptation of ideas presented in Porter.

46. An adaptation and summary of ideas presented by Henderson, Bruce B. *Henderson on Corporate Strategy.* Cambridge, MA: Abt Books, 1979, pp. 29-31.

47. This notion of defensive strategy was brought to the authors' attention by Ira H. Schlezinger, director of planning, Hillcrest Medical Center, Tulsa, OK.

48. Porter, Michael E. *Competitive Strategy: Techniques for Analyzing Industries and Competitors.* New York City: The Free Press, 1980, pp. 100-2. For a hard-line business approach to competitive strategy, see Henderson, Bruce D. *Henderson on Corporate Strategy.* Cambridge, MA: Abt Books, 1978, pp. 27-31, and 89-113.

49. Stromberg, Ross E. Handout for seminar given by Hanson, Bridgett, Marcus, Vlahos & Stromberg, San Francisco.

50. Stromberg, Ross E. Legal Issues for Diversification and Divesture, presented at Society for Hospital Planning of the American Hospital Association Seminar on Strategies for Hospital Diversification, Feb. 25, 1981. For more on this subject see Greenberg, Larry, and others. Organizational options: corporate reorganization. In: Minnesota Hospital Association, pp. 187-92; also, Hatfield II, John N. Restructuring: a responsible alternative to hospital closure. *Trustee.* 33:33, Dec. 1980; DeWitt, Cynthia. Getting down to business. *Trustee.* 34:21, Oct. 1981; Caldwell, G. B. Corporate restructuring: a special concern for the church hospital. *Bulletin of the American Protestant Hospital Association.* 44:20, Winter 1981; and Walker, S. R. Corporate restructuring: walk before you run. *Trustee.* 35:47, Sept. 1982.

Chapter 8

Strategic Choices: Values, Ethics, and Organizational Culture in the Strategic Management Process

"In any event, thinking about strategy, complexity, and incompleteness delves into a domain where one's personal beliefs, values, preferences, and expectations can have the most influence."

—Robert Kirk Mueller, *The Incompleat Board: The Unfolding of Corporate Governance*[1]

"Change implies an intervention in a complex web of past and present relations which have emerged in an evolving environment of values, understandings, agreements, and problem resolutions. Planning which ignores these relationships necessarily engenders resistances, hostilities, and blocking behavior. Even if these are forcibly overcome, there remains a residue of resistant feeling. Implementation fails as participants cling in varying degrees to previous identifications."

—Richard S. Bolan, *Planning in America: Learning from Turbulence*[2]

"Not everything at hand belongs in the future—make some important choices."

—Chinese fortune cookie

Once the various strategic alternatives that are open to an institution have been identified, its management faces the challenging task of deciding which strategies offer the most promising directions for the future. As with so much of life, strategy depends on knowing how to choose well; however, making a good choice is seldom easy. It is particularly difficult when the choice involves selecting the best option to guide an organization as complex and as socially relevant as the modern hospital. Not only must the choice be rational in the sense that it can lead to a desired outcome, but also in that it is suited to the values of the persons involved and to the *ethos* of the organization. At most, the alternative selected should do only minimal harm to both. For these reasons, strategic choices are often simultaneously the most systematic and the most human elements in the strategic management process.

The Elements of a Good Choice

"Making good choices depends on three elements: the quality of our *definition* of specific factors that must be satisfied, the quality of our *evaluations* of the available alternatives, and the quality of our *understanding* of what those alternatives can produce—for better or worse. . . . A good decision can only be made in the context of *what it is that needs to be accomplished.* No alternative is any better than its ability to do the job that needs to be done."
—Charles H. Kepner and
Benjamin B. Tregoe, *The New Rational Manager*[3]

Few alternatives fulfill all of management's expectations without presenting some new difficulties and risks. A diversification strategy that focuses on new programs for the aged may, for example, jeopardize a hospital's well being because of inadequate third-party reimbursement for long-term care services. Or, needed growth may require heavy borrowing at excessively high interest rates, which could financially overburden the institution for many years. *Therefore in selecting among several alternatives, management must decide which option will best meet its desired objectives with the fewest and most acceptable risks or adverse consequences.* Even if only one alternative is put forth, management must still determine whether it meets these requirements.[4]

William F. Glueck outlines four basic managerial factors that are helpful in understanding strategic choice decisions:[5]

Managerial perceptions of the organization's dependence on the external environment. Organizations do not operate in isolation. They depend on other individuals and units, such as owners, competitors, suppliers, customers, stakeholders, government, and community, for survival and success. In addition, hospitals rely on physicians and other health professionals without whom they would be unable to provide essential curative and diagnostic services. Except in crisis situations, a hospital's range of strategic choices is usually limited by its dependency on these groups. As a result, many of a hospital's strategies are *negotiated outcomes,* reflecting the different interests, needs, and expectations of many elements about which its management has little say.

Managerial attitudes toward risk. How much risk a hospital's leaders are willing to accept is an important determinant of its strategy. Some risk is inherent in every strategic decision because, as noted previously in this book, strategy always deals with an uncertain future. However, managers vary in their responses toward risk; so, too, do the other stakeholders who have a voice in what the institution does or proposes to do. Some people regard risk as necessary for success and are able to tolerate high-risk situations. Some try to hedge by balancing high-risk with low-risk choices. Others are inherently cautious and shy away from risk. To borrow the advice of Balthasar Gracian, a 17th-century sage, a strategist would do well to recognize that folly is always bold, but that a grain of boldness is an asset in dealing with worldly affairs, especially if one is able to cultivate "the art of being lucky."[6]

Managerial awareness of previous strategies. Past strategies can be either starting points or constraints in selecting new strategies. If known, they may sometimes even eliminate the need to develop a new strategy. The possibility of management being unaware of past strategies may seem odd, but hospital management in particular has rarely thought in strategic terms. Although the institution may have a sense of direction and pursue certain strategies, these are usually not expressed in written form nor are they necessarily consciously known either to the governing board or management. However, it is important to recognize that new strategies can evolve from past strategies and, further, that new strategies are often grafted to old strategies to accommodate changing conditions (see chapter 3).

Managerial power relationships and organizational structure. Organizational power relationships play an obvious role in strategic choices as they do in virtually all aspects of institutional management. Personality conflicts, jealousies, power plays, office politics, cliques, and other less-than-inspiring realities of organizational life not only influence choices, but also can determine the range of possible alternatives for consideration.

Five Decision Situations Confronting the Strategist

1. **The outcomes are certain.** The action leads to a single known outcome: Action 1 (A_1) results in Outcome 1 (O_1), A_2 in O_2, and so forth. Here, the decision maker has complete control of the outcome. Knowing which action or option leads to which outcome enables the decision maker to select the one that leads to the most preferred outcome.
2. **The outcomes are risky.** Action A_1 may lead to any one of a specified set of outcomes, for example, O_2, O_5, or O_{14}, but the decision maker is able to determine the probability of each outcome in the set. Determining which is the best alternative requires some notion of what is meant by best, because some possible outcomes are better than others associated with another course of action, and some are worse.
3. **The outcomes are partially controlled by another.** Is anyone else able to select or control the actual outcomes from among the possible ones associated with a given action (decision)? Here, the crucial factor is whether the other party has also assigned utilities to the outcomes, and, if so, what these utilities are. In a zero-sum game (one wins, one loses), the aim is to mix strategies to confound the opponent, who in discerning the strategy can take certain actions that can control or divert the outcome.
4. **The outcomes are messy.** A_1 is selected, but unexpected O_8 results, either because the decision maker does not understand the complex, nonlinear, multiple-loop structure of the underlying system or because he is not aware of the remarkable insensitivity to change of some of the system parameters. Many social planning ventures take place under these conditions. See works of Professor Jay W. Forrester, Massachusetts Institute of Technology, for more on this subject.
5. **The outcomes are unknown.** Unlike situations under risk, probabilities cannot be assigned to outcomes that are unknown. At best, the strategist can forecast a variety of outcomes based on certain assumptions, or he can "hang loose" and forget the situation entirely.

—Adapted from Anatol Rapaport,
Strategy and Conscience[7]

Strategic decisions perhaps would be less painful if proposed strategies could be divorced from individual sponsorship. But this is not possible in most management situations. Often a chain of successive sponsorships allows individuals to convince their superiors or colleagues of the desirability of certain actions. This internal movement and filtering of ideas through an organization may lead to competition among employees and staff, which can be good or bad, depending on the circumstances. However, when mistakes are made, a powerful person can shift the blame to others, creating resentments and, even worse, provoking fear of failure among subordinates, which can discourage new ideas or risk taking. Employees are well aware that, at times, even a small failure can wipe out big successes of the past. Therefore, low-level or middle managers are often reluctant to suggest strategic options that have little chance of approval or that might jeopardize their jobs.

As with all decisions, the choice of a strategy is made in the context of the persons involved and the particular strategic situation. The following quick checks place the options within the specific context and, therefore, are useful in comparing and choosing among competing alternatives:

- Consistency with overall mission and basic goals of the institution
- Consistency with past strategies
- Feasibility of accomplishing desired purpose
- Effectiveness in accomplishing results sought
- Consistency with managerial expectations or values
- Workability in terms of available or anticipated resource competencies
- Satisfactory (acceptable) degree of risk
- Acceptability to various stakeholder groups

- Flexibility in meeting demands of a volatile market
- Consistency or relevance to environmental or community changes or needs
- Cost-effectiveness
- Appropriate time horizon
- Compatability with organizational structure and culture
- Compatability with society goals and ethical values

These checks can be summarized in two basic questions: *Will the strategic alternative work? Is it the right thing to do?* The issue of workability is often determined by the availability and deployment of resources and predictable outcomes.[8] The rightness of a proposed strategic alternative involves such human constructions as personal preferences, ideals, ethics, organizational values, and societal consequences.

It is here that stakeholder concerns often surface. In chapter 4, mention was made of the importance of various groups inside and outside the institution—stakeholders—who have an interest in or voice in the institution's affairs and who may be affected by what the institution does or fails to do. In some instances, various groups may also have a vested interest in a proposed strategy, and its eventual success or failure depends on how well the strategy satisfies their interests or meets their expectations. As it is not always feasible to determine the groups' reactions in advance, assumptions about their behavior toward a proposed strategy or plan can be made and analyzed. Here are some prompting questions that may be helpful:[9]

- What assumptions are being made about a particular stakeholder group and its future behavior for the proposed strategy or plan to be successful?
- What are some counter assumptions? Do they have a significant impact on the choice of strategy or on the success of the strategy?
- Are there any "low probability, high-risk" stakeholders, that is, groups that are remote, easily overlooked, and usually unlikely to affect a strategy or a plan, but should they become active, can have an immense impact—either favorable or unfavorable—on the strategy or the plan?

Hospitals are basic sustenance organizations rooted in a long tradition of humanitarianism and community service.[10] Many who work in hospitals or who treat their patients are members of professional groups with equally long traditions and human concerns. Combined, these two overlapping value systems have set hospitals apart from other enterprises. These circumstances tend to make the hospital industry more cooperative than, for example, the garment industry, which is perceived as a cut-throat operation, or the merchandising field, in which competitors vie for market and price advantages.[11] These values also make hospital management cautious and hesitant to explore strategies that other organizations have found advantageous. Few hospital personnel, particularly those who carry the burden of devising institutional strategies, will argue with Cunningham's admonition that "There are business, professional, social, and moral values to be contemplated in all important hospital decisions and no computers or formulas to provide the answers."[12]

Thus, the strategy set of a hospital is molded by the values and personal traits of the persons who make the strategic choices. These persons view the various options open to them with acquired habits of thinking and with varying backgrounds, training, experiences, perceptions, beliefs, values, standards, expectations, and other personal traits that affect their decisions and actions.

Some alternatives seem more attractive than others for reasons other than their workability. They are considered the right thing to do, the actions that the organization *should* take, in the opinion of the chooser, to meet perceived obligations and goals. Developing a hospice program or a home health service appeals to the humanitarian values of one hospital's governing board. Offering high income and loan guarantees as inducements in recruiting physicians to staff satellite clinics whets the competitive appetites of another hospital's leaders. Terminating an unprofitable hospital-based skilled nursing facility does not trouble a board that measures success by bottom line financial results. Forging collaborative arrangements with other local hospitals makes good sense to hospital management accustomed to weighing its decisions in terms of community benefits. And corporate restructuring is viewed as an innovative strategy by a hospital eager to capitalize on new opportunities by diversifying its services.

Other alternatives seem to be clearly undesirable. They may simply be too risky for management, or they may be regarded as unprofitable, unworkable, unmanageable, or in other ways disadvantageous to the institution or inimical to its corporate beliefs. For example, abortion and family planning services are out of the question for many church-sponsored hospitals. A proposal to grant staff privileges to osteopathic physicians (or to allopathic physicians at an osteopathic hospital) to bolster admissions may be contrary to a hospital's past policies or unacceptable to its medical staff. Employing full-time, salaried physicians to head clinical services is anathema to the attending staffs at some hospitals. Admitting uncompensated care patients may be viewed as suicidal by the governing boards of institutions with limited access to philanthropic support to underwrite resulting losses. Joint planning with neighboring hospitals may be summarily dismissed as a "pipe dream" by institutions with long histories of noncooperation or antagonism. The recognition that some hospitals do provide family planning services, have joint staffs involving the two schools of medicine, employ full-time chiefs of clinical services, treat substantial numbers of uncompensated care patients, and that, increasingly, many hospitals nationwide are planning and working together to improve services to their communities simply emphasizes the point that these decisions are made in the context of the persons involved and that these, in turn, often reflect the beliefs and traditions that form the basis of the institution's culture.

Despite many difficulties and value differences, choices are made and new strategies are devised. However, many of the strategic choices made by institutions are merely extensions of past experiences rather than products of future-focused thinking. Their leaders have learned to think in practical terms: because an idea worked yesterday, it will work with equal success tomorrow. Thus, they base today's choices on yesterday's successes. In less turbulent times, when change was slower and less pervasive, this experience was a reasonable basis for making choices. It may be a dangerous way of doing so today.[13]

Could This Be Your Organization?

"The intrinsic difficulty of determining and choosing among strategic alternatives leads many companies to do what the rest of the industry is doing rather than to make an independent determination of opportunity and resources. Sometimes the companies of an industry run like sheep all in one direction. The similarity among the strategies, at least in some periods of history, of insurance companies, banks, railroads, and airplane manufacturers may lead one to ask whether strategic decisions were based upon industry convention or upon independent analysis. Whether the similarity of timing, decision, and reaction to competition constitutes independent appraisals of each company's situation, or whether imitation took the place of independent decision is the basis of some wonder. At any rate, the similarity of one company's strategy to that of its competitors does not constitute the assurance of soundness which it might at first suggest."
—Kenneth R. Andrews, *The Concept of Corporate Strategy*[14]

Executives in many types of enterprises are learning, often to their dismay, that even a good strategy can fail for reasons unrelated to its workability or consistency to an organization's overall mission and goals. If a strategy is not clearly understood by those who are expected to carry it out, if it is contrary to corporate values and traditions, if it violates employees' basic beliefs, or if it departs radically from established ways of company behavior, it can fail. Indeed, these shared values and beliefs that constitute the organization's culture can be major assets when they are consistent with proposed strategy; otherwise they are almost insurmountable barriers when they do not mesh with the new strategy.[15]

As with all human organizations, hospitals have distinct personalities that differ from each other in important ways. These differences both shape and limit what they do and what they aspire to do. More important, they determine how the institution operates—its style—and how it intends to confront the future—its strategy. Some hospitals are highly structured organizations, with formal, "tight" management styles that emphasize stern lines of authority, management-by-objectives, and clear-cut standard operating procedures. Their strategies are likely to be equally formed and well honed. Other hospitals are easy going, slow paced, "homey" institutions that radiate a friendly concern for patients, employees, and visitors. It is unlikely that they would elect to follow aggressive marketing strategies or introduce tight management and fiscal controls. Other hospitals are physician dominated and this, in turn, influences their choice of strategies. Some hospitals are obviously community-centered enterprises. They search for new service opportunities and new constituencies. They are often the pace-setting medical care institutions in their communities.

These corporate personalities and resulting behavior patterns are shaped over time by management. By example and edict certain values are instilled in employees and passed down to succeeding generations of workers. It is easy to understand why these traditions are not easy to change and how they can influence future strategies.

Three Strategic Postures for Hospitals

"The most successful strategies turn out to be clusters of strategies in support of a particular goal. . . . The strategic position established for any one goal may vary according to the particular strategy of the institution. Generally, there are three positions or postures that an institution may wish to establish—a superiority position, an equivalency position, or an inferiority position.

"A strategic superiority position implies that the institution is willing to provide sufficient resources to maintain a competitively superior position in an attempt to reach a goal. This position is generally taken when goals are established that pursue new, improved, and expanded services. The position does not imply superiority at all costs, but it does imply that sufficient resources will be expanded to gain a specific position.

"A strategic equivalency position implies that plans are developed that would place the institution in a similar position in terms of competitive thrust to a position it previously held. Essentially, this position indicates that ground will not be lost in seeking a particular goal. It implies an adequate amount of resources to develop the goal.

"A strategic inferiority position implies that the institution is willing to sacrifice its position in pursuit of certain goals and to accept a position of inferiority in certain areas that do not present optimal challenges or impose severe threats."
—William J. Bodzek, *Hospitals*[16]

All organizations are responsible for the social consequences of their actions and, to a lesser extent, are held accountable for transactions that violate prevailing ethical codes of the societies in which they operate. Because of the nature of their services and their unique role in society, hospitals are expected to adhere to higher standards in these respects than business firms and other less altruistic endeavors. As Cunningham has happily observed, "It is to their credit that [hospital trustees] do use a different value system in the hospital board-room" than in their business environments.[17]

Although a clear consensus on specific social responsibilities of business doesn't exist in business,[18] such a consensus does exist among hospitals. In 1981, the American Hospital Association Board of Trustees approved a set of guidelines on ethical conduct and relationships for health care institutions. Despite some uncertainties such as the recent interest in market forces and the impact of competition on the delivery of health services, these guidelines continue to be useful to trustees and others responsible for shaping hospital strategies and policies.

In addition to management, medical staff, and employees, a proposed strategy must be also acceptable to an institution's other stakeholders and to outside community interests. Hospitals are learning, for example, that they cannot afford to be bad neighbors. They are expected to act as responsible and enlightened property owners, to be good employers, to be fair in their business dealings, and to carry out the obligations of a socially responsible institution. They do not have license to act against broader community interests, however noble or justifiable the cause may seem to management. For example, in the past, some hospitals were amazed to discover that their presumed well-reasoned and well-intended plans for expanding services to their communities were angrily denounced by those same communities as poorly conceived and self-serving to institutional interests. Although the issue of community participation and control in hospital affairs has diminished since the early 1970s, hospitals are still well advised to reflect seriously and act positively on their obligations to the communities they aspire to serve.

Forging New Coalitions for Change

"One step in bringing about change, on almost any scale, is to create a shared body of values, attitudes, or experiences, a new 'membership' in which individuals reinforce one another in using, extending, or defending a new idea against the pull of inertia, reluctance, or outright opposition."
—Nancy Foy, *The Yin and Yang of Organizations*[19]

A hospital's leaders must make choices that strike a balance between the institution's perceived opportunities and its competencies and resources, without losing sight of personal values and entrenched corporate beliefs and traditions. This chapter has discussed some of the obvious requirements and restrictions in making these choices.[20] In the final analysis, this is all that it can do. It cannot determine the choices that the strategist will make in real life. However, these thoughtful words may dissuade readers from becoming discouraged:

"Whenever choice is compounded of rational analysis which can have more than one outcome, of aspiration and desire which can run the whole range of human ambition, and a sense of responsibility which changes the appeal of alternatives, it cannot be reduced to quantitative approaches or to the exactness which management science can apply to narrower questions. Managers contemplating strategic decisions must be willing to make them without the guidance of rules, with confidence in their own judgment, which will have been seasoned by repeated analysis of similar questions. They must be aware that more than one decision is possible and that they are not seeking the single right answer. They can take encouragement from the fact that the manner in which an organization implements the chosen program can help to validate the original decision. . . . The final decision, which should be made as deliberately as possible after a detailed consideration of the issues we have attempted to separate, is an act of will and desire as much as of intellect."[21]

American Hospital Association Guidelines on Ethical Conduct and Relationships for Health Care Institutions

These guidelines were developed originally in 1973 by the Special Committee on Ethics of the AHA Council on Management and Planning. They were approved by the Board of Trustees in 1974 for publication by the American College of Hospital Administrators (ACHA) in its pamphlet titled Code of Ethics. *In view of the increasing accountability of health care institutions to their communities, the guidelines were revised and updated in 1980 by the Council on Management and approved by the General Council.*

Health care institutions are service organizations that provide patient care and a varying range of education, research, public health, and social services for their communities. These institutions carry public responsibilities for their own conduct, the health care of their patients, and the health of their communities. This role places special obligations upon health care institutions and their representatives to adhere to ethical principles of conduct. The following guidelines are intended to assist members of the American Hospital Association in defining their institutional policies, ethical relationships, and practices.

- Health care institutions should be interested in the overall health status of people in addition to providing direct patient care services.
- The public has accorded high priority to the availability of services to the sick and injured, but there are limits to the individual and collective resources available for this purpose. Recognizing this, health care institutions should support the most effective use of economic and other resources to ensure access to comprehensive services of high quality.
- The community's health objectives are advanced when all health care providers and social, welfare, educational, and other agencies work together in planning and offering improved services. Health care institutions should promote and support such cooperation.*
- Patient care services are inherently personal in nature. Health care institutions should maintain organizational relationships, policies, and systems that are conducive to humane and individualized care for those being served.
- Health care institutions, wherever possible and consistent with ethical commitments of the institution, should ensure respect and consideration for the dignity and individuality of patients, employees, physicians, and others.

- Health care institutions should establish and maintain internal policies, practices, standards of performance, and systematic methods of evaluation that emphasize high quality, safety, and effectiveness of care.
- Health care institutions, being dependent upon community confidence and support, should accept an ethical sense of public accountability; reflect fairness, honesty, and impartiality in all activities and relationships; manage their resources prudently; and ensure that reports to the public are factual and clear in interpreting institutional goals, status, and accomplishments.
- Health care institutions should relate to their communities and to each other constructively and in ways that merit and preserve public confidence in them, both individually and collectively.
- Health care institutions that operate on a nonprofit basis should feel free to publicize their various tax-exempt purposes that are deserving of charitable and philanthropic support.** This may include an ongoing program of public relations and may range from reminders of the opportunities for memorials and charitable bequests to the conducting of a fund drive for a particular purpose. In responding to charitable and philanthropic interests or in soliciting contributions, health care institutions should not capitalize on the sensitivities of individuals in any way that might subject the institution's motivations to ethical criticism. Likewise, in directing such publicity to those who may be in the chain of providing goods and services to the institution, care should be taken to ensure that the institution's approach complies with any legal restrictions on this activity,† does not suggest a relation to patronage that would support adverse reimbursement consequences, and precludes any suggestion that future patronage by the institution would be affected by charitable or philanthropic generosity. The demonstration of ethical commitment by the health care institution may well be the strongest assurance of continued charitable and philanthropic support.

References

*See *Statement on Health Planning.* AHA no. S025, 1976.

**See *Guidelines on Advertising by Hospitals.* AHA no. G030, 1977.

†Review should be made of possible technical violations of the Medicare-Medicaid Anti-Fraud and Abuse Act (P.L. 95-142) and similar legislation. Also see *Guidelines on Resolution of Conflicts of Interest in Health Care Institutions.* AHA no. G004, 1975.

Notes

1. Mueller, Robert Kirk. *The Incompleat Board: The Unfolding of Corporate Governance.* Lexington, MA: D. C. Heath and Company, 1981, p. 11.

2. Bolan, Richard S. Mapping the planning theory terrain. In: Godschalk, David R., editor. *Planning in America: Learning from Turbulence.* Washington, DC: American Institute of Planners, 1974, pp. 31-2.

3. Kepner, Charles H., and Tregoe, Benjamin B. *The New Rational Manager.* Princeton, NJ: Princeton University Press, 1981, pp. 85-6.

4. For more on the general subject of making choices and the thinking pattern for making them, see Kepner and Tregoe, chapters 4 and 5.

5. Glueck, William F. *Strategic Management and Business Policy.* New York City: McGraw-Hill Book Co., 1980, pp. 281-84.

6. Gracian, Balthasar. *The Art of Worldly Wisdom.* Translated from the Spanish by Joseph Jacobs. New York City: The Macmillan Company, 1955, pp. 12, 45, 57, and 107. This *vade mecum* (also known as *Gracian's Manual)* has been translated into several languages and reprinted in many editions since its first publication in 1647 in Spain. It is a little gem that will delight anyone who must grapple with the affairs of the world. Despite its many reprintings, it is not easily obtainable, but acquiring it is well worth the effort. For more on opportunities and risks, see Drucker, Peter F. *Managing for Results.* London: Pan Books, Ltd., 1967, chapter 13.

7. An elaboration and adaptation of a list prepared by Rapaport, Anatol. *Strategy and Conscience.* New York City: Harper and Row, 1964.

8. See Rumelt, Richard P. Evaluation of strategy: theory and models. In: Schendel, Dan E., and Hofer, Charles W., editors. *Strategic Management: A New View of Business Policy and Planning.* Boston: Little, Brown and Company, 1979, pp. 199 ff.

9. These questions are adapted from Mason, Richard O., and Mitroff, Ian L. *Challenging Strategic Planning Assumptions: Theory, Cases, and Techniques.* New York City: John Wiley and Sons, 1981, pp. 98-101.

10. For more on the hospital as a sustenance organization (institution that society has organized to enable its members to survive), see Peters, Joseph P., and Haldeman, M.D., Jack C., Areawide planning of hospitals and related medical care facilities. In DeGroot, M.D., Leslie J., compiler. *Medical Care: Social and Organization Aspects.* Springfield, IL: Charles C Thomas, Publisher, 1966.

11. For more on the subject of industrial values, see Rothschild, William E. *Putting It All Together: A Guide to Strategic Thinking.* New York City: AMACOM, 1976, p. 74.

12. Cunningham Jr., Robert M. It's a question of ethics. *Trustee.* 53:36, Dec. 1979.

13. See Ewalt Jr., William R. Foreword. In: Skibbins, G. J. *Organizational Evolution: A Program for Managing Radical Change.* New York City: AMACOM, 1974.

14. Andrews, Kenneth R. *The Concept of Corporate Strategy.* Homewood, IL: Richard D. Irwin, Inc., 1980, pp. 43-4.

15. Corporate culture: the hard-to-change values that spell success or failure. *Business Week.* 2660:148, Oct. 27, 1980.

16. Bodzek, J. William. Corporate approach lends controls over complex environment. *Hospitals, J.A.H.A.* 53:71, Nov. 1, 1979.

17. Cunningham, p. 37.

18. Jackson Jr., Donald W., and Aldag, Ramon J. Planning for corporate social actions. *Managerial Planning.* 29:28, Sept.-Oct. 1980.

19. Foy, Nancy. *The Yin and Yang of Organizations.* New York City: William Morrow and Company, Inc., 1980, p. 181.

20. For more on this important subject, see Peters, Joseph P., and Wacker, Ronald C. Hospital strategic planning must be rooted in values and ethics. *Hospitals.* 56:90, June 16, 1982.

21. Andrews, pp. 102-4.

Chapter 9
The Strategic Planning Retreat

"To change things in a group or organization, you often need to build a critical mass of people who agree with you and each other that the change is vital and positive. One way to get that critical mass quickly and easily is to start with a small, clearly identified group, whose members already look to one another as people of sound, wise views."

—Nancy Foy, *The Yin and Yang of Organizations*[1]

"The grouping of 'things' (in the widest sense) is the most basic and necessary element of our perception and conception of reality. While it is obvious that no two things will ever be exactly alike, the ordering of the world into (complexly intersecting and overlapping) groups composed of members which all share an important element in common gives structure to what would otherwise be a phantasmagoric chaos."

—Paul Watzlawick and others, *Change: Principles of Problem Formation and Problem Resolution*[2]

"Change is a contest: but it is that kind of contest which can easily become a fight, in which more and more social resources are consumed to the point where the outcome can only be a loss for both sides. Men destroy themselves not always because they have to in order to defend a principle, but sometimes merely because they have not learned how to communicate through confrontations and how to keep their encounters socially inexpensive."

—F. G. Bailey, *Stratagems and Spoils: A Social Anthropology of Politics*[3]

Strategic thinking is essentially a do-it-yourself activity. Experience indicates that the best way to begin is to convene a group of knowledgeable persons—the best thinkers—in a congenial environment away from their usual place of business to participate in carefully prepared, structured work sessions. These sessions are popularly known in management circles as *retreats,* because they force the participants to turn away, to retreat, from preoccupations with day-to-day concerns and to focus their attention on long-term issues and problems.[4] Thus, a retreat is a period, usually one or two days, in which the participants are guided through concentrated task-oriented and social activities. Its goal is to improve the effectiveness of the participants in interacting with each other and working with the matters under consideration. Its effectiveness is measured by how well the group is able to reach a consensus about future actions.

There are many types of management retreats. Some are designed to convey knowledge, some emphasize skill-building, some focus on solving problems, some aspire to resolve concerns or to facilitate discussion of issues that seem to hinder effectiveness, and some are meant to renew commitment, usually by emphasizing social interaction and presenting awards for outstanding performance and dedication.[5] A management retreat that has been gaining wide acceptance in hospital circles in recent years is the *strategic planning retreat, strategic retreat, or, simply, planning retreat.* It is designed to identify outside change and the organization's ability to manage it.

A hospital can elect to have its own staff organize and carry out a strategic planning retreat, or it can employ an outside consultant or a consulting firm to provide these services. Of course, published information can be relied on for guidelines.[6] No matter who organizes and implements the retreat, certain decisions or tasks must be made or performed for the retreat to be operational and successful: gaining acceptance of the idea, using outside versus in-house resources, identifying the participants, selecting a suitable locale, determining the duration and the time of week, establishing a balance between process and content, and following up after the session.

Gaining acceptance. Even though a hospital already may be carrying out an organized long-range planning venture, its management may not be aware that something more is required. Many hospital leaders equate planning with the construction of facilities, the acquisition of new equipment, or the preparation of capital and operating budgets. An outsider, a new board member, or a change in top management may be required to convince them that deeper probing of external change and internal capabilities is necessary for the institution's survival. A strategic planning retreat can be a very effective way of stimulating such probings. But, convincing a hospital's leaders that the required expenditures of time and money (retreats can be costly in terms of both) are necessary and productive can be difficult.

Instead, someone in top management or at the board level usually perceives a need for new strategies and convinces a few key colleagues who, in turn, convince others. They may turn to an outside consultant who advises them that a retreat is the best way to launch a strategic planning endeavor. The consultant is then asked to assist in making the necessary arrangements and to conduct the retreat. Or, management may request a member of its staff to do this.

The key is, of course, that someone is able to sell the idea of a retreat and that sufficient commitment and enthusiasm are aroused to carry out the idea. Therefore, when a hospital board agrees to underwrite such a retreat and the majority of those invited plan to attend, the venture is off to a good start. How successful it will prove to be depends on how well the various other tasks are performed.

Using outside versus in-house resources. Conducting a strategic retreat is a challenging endeavor. The participants must be guided through a process that enables them to identify and resolve issues, to focus their attention on an uncertain future, to work with intellectual abstractions whose practical values are not immediately evident, and to take a hard look at the institution's ability to deal with outside change. Some who attend are willing participators and contribute readily to the deliberations, others participate very little and must be drawn into the discussion. At least one is long-winded and expresses an opinion on almost every subject. A skilled retreat leader is able to handle these personality types and situations. A skilled retreat leader also knows how to move the deliberations toward the desired goals without the use of gimmickry and games that can alienate a sophisticated audience. An outsider who is not on intimate terms with the audience is usually better able to meet these challenges than a hospital staff member who works with the participants on a regular basis. However, an in-house planner or other member of the management team can conduct a good retreat. Many have done so successfully, because they have developed the necessary skills and know-how. A good rule is to employ outsiders if in-house capabilities are limited or if insiders, as familiar figures, would be unable to arouse the necessary enthusiasm or interest to keep the proceedings moving.

Identifying the participants. This decision is usually the most difficult in organizing a retreat. Ideally, invitations should be sent to only the 12 best thinkers, as suggested in chapter 2. However, most hospitals find this impractical, although they may be able to limit the participants in subsequent aspects of the strategic management process. Many hospitals elect to invite the entire board and interestingly, board members usually attend. The CEO and other members of the hospital's management team are also involved, both as participants and as resource staff.

What to Look for in Groups

"In all human interactions there are two major ingredients—content and process. The first deals with the subject matter on the task upon which the group is working. In most interactions, the focus of attentions of all persons is on the content. The second ingredient, process, is concerned with what is happening between and to group members while the group is working. Group process, or dynamics, deals with such items as morale, feeling, tone, atmosphere, influence, participation, styles of influence, leadership struggles, conflict, competition, cooperation, etc. In most interactions, very little attention is paid to process, even when it is the major cause of ineffective group action. Sensitivity to group process will better enable one to diagnose group problems early and deal with them more effectively. Since these processes are present in all groups, awareness of them will enhance a person's worth to a group and enable him to be a more effective group participant."

—J. W. Pfeiffer and
J. E. Jones, *The 1972 Handbook for Group Facilitators*[7]

Selected members of the medical staff should also be invited. Hospitals will vary in how they make these selections; many simply ask the president of the medical staff or the medical board to make the determination. Experience indicates that, for whatever reasons, medical staff attendance tends to be lower than for board members or administrative staff. Therefore, a few extra physicians should be invited as some of them may not be able to attend.

Selecting the locale. The worst place to conduct a retreat is at the hospital. Not only are many distractions possible, particularly to the physicians and administrative staff in attendance, but the arrangement itself lessens the importance of the event, giving it the impression of just another meeting. A remote hotel or resort is preferable because the participants are usually required to spend the night there and have opportunities to talk and otherwise interact at meals and social events. A high-quality resort atmosphere where golf, tennis, and other recreation is available adds an element of reward at little extra cost. A less preferable arrangement, although it is quite suitable for a one-day session, is a downtown hotel or a nearby country club.

Determining the duration and the time of week. A one-day retreat is easiest to sell, but has the least emotional impact. Two full days is the best arrangement, but may be too long for many persons. One and a half days seems to be the most successful option: it draws the best attendance and still allows a desired balance of work sessions and social interaction. A longer session can be developed, preferably over a weekend, if sufficient free time is assigned for recreation or rest.

The time of week is also important, with a late Friday afternoon through Saturday afternoon ranking as the most acceptable arrangement. Weekday sessions exclude those who cannot easily get off from work and may interfere with occupations in other ways. In addition, a series of weeknight sessions is wearying.

Making presession arrangements on essential details. Even if a consultant is hired to conduct the retreat, he will usually require hospital staff assistance to make various presession arrangements. Decisions must be made on such important items as duration, time, and place of the meeting; budget; participants; focus; and dozens of seemingly small, but nonetheless important, considerations. Letters of invitation, timing, dress, menus, entertainment, training aids (easels, blackboards, projectors, mark-

Agenda for Strategic Planning Retreat, 1 Day

8:15 a.m.	Coffee
8:30	Opening remarks, by chairman, Board of Trustees
8:35	Background observations and introduction of consultant by chairman, Capital Improvements and Planning Committee
8:45	Introduction to planning and the planning climate: "As We Face The Future"(consultant)
10:15	Break
10:30	Work group sessions on situation analysis
12:00 noon	Lunch
1:00 p.m.	Group reports
2:30	Break
2:45	Suggestions for action: "Where Do We Go From Here" (consultant)
4:45	Concluding Remarks, by chairman, Capital Improvements and Planning Committee

Agenda for Strategic Planning Retreat, 1½ Days

Friday

4:00 p.m.	Introductory remarks
4:30	Review of current strategy
5:30	Break
5:45	Review of current mission/basic beliefs
7:00	Reception followed by dinner

Saturday

8:00 a.m.	Summary of previous sessions
8:15	Environmental assessment
9:30	Break
9:45	Stakeholder analysis: who do we really serve?
10:30	Assessment of present and future capabilities/resources
11:45	Lunch
1:00 p.m.	Identification of key issues: triggers for change
1:30	Some options for the future
2:30	Break
2:45	Choice of future directions/strategy and guidelines for action
4:00	Next steps
4:30	Adjourn

Agenda for Strategy Development Retreat, 2½ Days

Wednesday

6:00 p.m.	Reception
6:45	Dinner
8:10	Introductory remarks
8:20	Retreat overview
8:30	Introduction to strategy
8:45	Environmental assessment (group discussion)

Thursday

8:00 a.m.	Breakfast
9:00	Current beliefs
10:30	Break
10:45	Stakeholder analysis
12:30 p.m.	Lunch
1:30	Current resources and future capabilities
3:00	Break
3:15	Alternative strategies
5:30	Break
6:00	Reception
6:45	Dinner

Friday

8:00 a.m.	Breakfast
9:00	Testing of alternatives
10:30	Break
10:45	Choice and specification of future direction
12:30 p.m.	Lunch
1:30	Articulation of direction
3:00	Break
3:15	Next steps
4:00	Adjourn

Agenda for a Weekend Retreat, with Time Allocated for Recreation, 2½ Days*

Friday

12:00 noon	Lunch
1:00 p.m.	Introductory remarks: introduction to strategy
2:00	Who we are/what we believe in/where we are headed
3:00	Break
3:15-5:30	Continuation of above
6:20	Reception followed by dinner

Saturday

7:00 a.m.	Breakfast
8:00	Review of previous sessions
8:15	Environmental assessment
9:45	Break
10:00	Stakeholder analysis
11:00	Assessment of present and future capabilities/resources
12:00 noon	Free time for recreation
5:00-6:30 p.m.	Identificaton of key issues/triggers for change
7:00	Dinner

Sunday

8:00 a.m.	New directions/strategies/guidelines for future action
9:45	Break
10:00	Where do we go from here?
11:00	Brunch
12:00 noon	Adjourn

*If recreational time is omitted, this can be reduced to two days.

ing pens, and other items used by the retreat leader), meeting room set-up arrangements, name tags, preparation and distribution of hand-out materials, recreation and social events for spouses (if invited), between-session or during-session refreshments, billing for unrelated expenses (such as bar bills and gift shop purchases), and check-out time are such considerations.

In addition, someone in administration must work with the consultant or retreat leader to reserve a block of hotel rooms and appropriate conference and meeting rooms and to handle necessary financial arrangements. Staff must also be made available before and during the retreat to resolve problems, take messages, supervise meeting arrangements, record minutes, answer questions about schedules and accommodations, and carry out various supporting tasks. Sufficient advance preparation time—certainly not less than a month and preferably more—should be allowed to make these arrangements.

Establishing a balance between content and focus. Unfocused, smorgasbord-type retreats result in dissatisfaction and cause some participants to wonder why they came. It is the easiest type of retreat to arrange because there are few tough choices on what to offer and what not to offer. Thematic retreats with a tightly defined focus and structured questionings and discussions are more likely to develop into productive results, especially if conducted by an experienced leader. A suggested agenda for a strategic retreat is (1) identification and analysis of emerging issues (outside-in, analysis of competition, stakeholder analysis); (2) appraisal of implications or impacts of these emerging issues on the institution and how they will affect or be affected by its shared basic beliefs and values; (3) development of alternative means of dealing with these issues; (4) choice; and (5) future determination of strategies. Considering all of these topics in depth in a one-day meeting is obviously impractical; however, identifying three or four major external developments and their future impact on the institution and proposing tentative strategies should be possible at such a meeting.

Skilled group session leaders sometimes rely on a GAIA (God, ain't it awful) approach to stimulate comments on what's going on out there. This is done by asking the participants to identify some GAIA developments that promise to impact unfavorably on the organization. The approach works equally well with conservatives or liberals, as anyone can regard undesirable situations as fiendish conspiracies by those who disagree with their points of view. In any event, it is almost a sure-fire technique for getting the participants at a retreat or committee meeting to talk about environmental threats and challenges.[8]

Avoiding some common traps at retreats. The manner in which a retreat is conducted or organized can have a direct effect on its success. The following arrangements are common mistakes that should be avoided:

- If the chairman or retreat leader has the only copy of the agenda, no one else knows what to expect. Therefore, it is difficult for participants to feel involved.
- A formal classroom-style seating arrangement (row of chairs facing the front) discourages participation and gives a nonverbal clue that all action and wisdom originates in the front of the room, from the teacher. An open U-shape arrangement works best in groups of under 30.
- Long introduction of speakers produces a psychological distance between the speakers and the participants. If an extensive introduction is required, an appropriate curriculum vitae or biographical listing should be prepared and distributed as a handout to the audience at the beginning of the meeting.
- A coffee or other break should not be so prolonged that it wastes time or disrupts the continuity of the deliberations.
- A retreat is not the place to identify and discuss every threat or opportunity that the institution may face in the future. Therefore, retreat coordinators should avoid trying to do too much in a short time. Three or four key issues should be selected and a consensus on how to handle them should be reached.
- Neglecting to carry the group into the future can be very detrimental. Therefore, every meeting should end with a call for some future action to guarantee that the work of the meeting will pay off. Decisions and assignments should be made about who will do what and when, and a reporting system should be established. A summary report of the retreat should be prepared and distributed immediately following the last session.

Following up. A strategic retreat is simply a beginning point for the strategic management process. At best, the participants are able to design a strategy and identify major areas for future emphasis. These decisions must eventually be sharpened and submitted for board approval before they can be adopted as official hospital policy. Postsession follow-up begins with a written summary of the retreat that is sent to all participants, including those who were invited but were unable to attend. Subsequent actions will vary with the existing or proposed strategic planning structure and the organization's style in dealing with such matters.

The above advice does not necessarily reflect the opinion of other competent retreat leaders. One highly experienced planner and leader of retreats opens the proceedings with a case study, summarizing information about the case hospital and its community, programs, staff, and resources in approximately six pages. This exercise enables the participants to warm up on a real-life situation, thereby preparing them to review their own situation and concerns. With this tool, the leader is able to inaugurate a process that enables the participants to develop a *plan for planning,* which, among other things, reinforces the group's commitment to long-range planning, identifies the institution's strengths and weaknesses and the opportunities and threats that it faces in the future, highlights five or six big issues that should be addressed by the hospital in its future planning, reaffirms the charge to the long-range planning committee and establishes target dates and expected products. There is much merit in this approach, and some hospitals seem comfortable working within this framework. However, it involves long-range planning more than strategy formulation. As such, it does not go far enough in contributing toward a meaningful hospital strategic management process.

In summary, a well-designed, properly conducted strategic planning retreat that is held for one and a half to two days in a congenial setting, preferably at a distance from the hospital, has proven to be an effective way of developing new strategies and for getting a continuing strategic management process under way. With a skilled leader, not only is the event rewarding, it also can be fun.

Notes

1. Foy, Nancy. *The Yin and Yang of Organizations.* New York City: William Morrow and Company, Inc., 1980, p. 183.

2. Watzlawick, Paul, and others. *Change: Principles of Problem Formation and Problem Resolution.* New York City: W. W. Norton & Company, Inc., 1974, p. 4.

3. Bailey, F. G. *Stratagems and Spoils: A Social Anthropology of Politics.* New York City: Schocken Books, 1969, p. 224.

4. Retreats have been conducted for a long time by religious orders, especially by the Jesuits, to stimulate introspective self assessments through spiritual exercises in a quiet, unharried atmosphere for the spiritual betterment of the participants. A client organization labeled its recent one-day strategy work session an "advance" to reflect its president's hope that the session would advance the future progress of the institution.

5. For more on the various types of retreats and for specific advice on designing and managing them, see Webber, James B. *Designing a Board Retreat.* Report prepared for the Alpha Center for Health Planning, May 1979, and Sanderson, Bruce R. The whys and hows of a board retreat. *Trustee.* 32:51, Sept. 1979.

6. See Hardy, James M. *Corporate Planning for Nonprofit Organizations.* 1972 National YMCA Program Materials. New York City: Association Press, 1972.

7. Pfeiffer, J. W., and Jones, J. E. *The 1972 Handbook for Group Facilities.* vol. 11. La Jolla, CA: University Associates Publishers, 1972, p. 21.

8. An elaboration of an idea suggested by Kathleen D. Dannemiller, University of Michigan, Ann Arbor.

Chapter 10

Preparing for the Future: Real-Life Examples of Formal Strategies

"You have to take life as it happens, but you should try to make it happen the way you want to take it."

—An old German adage

"Being explicit about business definitions means, at a minimum, setting up *screening* procedures that channel an organization's growth into areas of maximum opportunity and comparative competitive advantage from an incremental *and* overall point of view."

—Derek F. Abell, *Defining The Business: The Starting Point of Strategic Planning*[1]

"One thorn of experience is worth a whole wilderness of warnings."

—David Campbell, Ph.D., *If You Don't Know Where You're Going, You'll Probably End Up Somewhere Else*[2]

"A strategy is a statement of an organization's investment priorities, the management thrust, and the ways that it will use its strengths and correct its limitations to pursue the opportunities and avoid the threats facing it. . . . The test of [its] soundness is whether a strategy is consistent with reality and feasible to implement."

—William E. Rothschild, *Putting It All Together: A Guide to Strategic Thinking*[3]

The preceding chapters have been intentionally prescriptive, presenting some general advice that will be useful to managers in a variety of hospital settings. This chapter follows a different approach. It describes two real-life situations that have been altered somewhat to maintain the institutions' anonymity. The strategies and guidelines developed by these are by no means designed to serve as prototypes. As with any real-life effort, they reflect the specific circumstances of the moment and the values of the participants, realities that usually cannot be repeated exactly in other hospital situations. Nonetheless, this material is useful for orientation to the process and the product and for analysis.

Some Thoughts to Remember

"Strategy is a human construction; it must in the long run be responsive to human needs. It must ultimately inspire commitment. It must stir an organization to successful striving against competition. Some people have to have their hearts in it."
—Kenneth R. Andrews, *The Concept of Corporate Strategy*[4]

General Hospital

General Hospital of Northeast Lincoln County is a 360-bed, voluntary general hospital offering an array of hospital inpatient and outpatient services to what is essentially a small city and a surrounding suburban population. In its general service area, there are several other large hospitals with an equal array of programs. This situation undoubtedly accounts for the emphasis on competitive strategies outlined here.

The following plan is the first attempt that General Hospital made to define its strategies in writing. Heretofore, its plans sprang from a simple mission statement that emphasized a comprehensive approach to local health care needs and specified a variety of acute short-term inpatient and related emergency and outpatient services. This mission was much too broad and too diffuse to provide real direction for future planning. With the help of an outside consultant to guide the hospital board of trustees and its Special Committee on Strategic Planning, a process similar to the plan outlined in this book was organized and implemented. A series of retreats and follow-up meetings was held during four months, with good participation by the board, the medical staff, and management. The product of these deliberations, the following strategic plan, is based on the findings and recommendations of the Special Committee on Strategic Planning as approved by the board of trustees. The plan is organized into the following major sections:

1. Introduction
2. Conclusions from environmental and comparative analyses
3. Basic beliefs
4. Strategy for markets and services
5. Guidelines for competing
6. Guidelines for implementation

1 . Introduction

The hospital's basic beliefs (section 3) are the foundation for choices made regarding the direction the hospital will take in terms of markets and services (section 4) and how these choices will be approached and carried out (sections 5 and 6). Section 2 shows the close relationship between the findings in sections 3 through 6 and the results of the environmental and comparative analyses. It also serves as a reminder that if significant changes take place in these external factors, adjustments in the strategic plan must be considered.

Several major themes provide focus and demonstrate the interrelationships among the many elements of the plan:

- General Hospital must maintain and, where appropriate, strengthen its current service and market positions and expand selectively and effectively into new markets.
- The hospital must adopt a more aggressive posture toward regulatory controls and a more competitive stance toward hospitals in its service area.

- The hospital must increase its capability to anticipate new developments in health care and changes in its external environment, to establish explicit direction and cohesion, and to implement new initiatives expeditiously.

2. Conclusions from environmental and comparative analyses

Various environmental factors and the actions of other local health providers will have a direct and major impact on the hospital's future role and direction. The most critical of these are as follows:

- Changes in the rate-setting and reimbursement system will probably benefit the hospital in the short run. However, stringent restrictions applied to patient service revenue will have a long-term negative effect on hospital finances.
- Planning and other regulatory controls will limit increases in inpatient costs and revenue by decreasing the number of hospital beds in the region, limiting the introduction of high-cost services and technology, promoting early detection and cost-effective alternatives to inpatient care, and applying more stringent utilization controls.
- Although the supply of physicians in the service area is likely to be adequate, attracting high-caliber physicians to the community will continue to be difficult.
- The age, ethnic composition, and health attitudes of the local population will continue to change, presenting opportunities and challenges for the hospital.
- The hospital industry in the region is consolidating, and the number and type of multi-institutional arrangements are expected to increase.
- The hospital will operate within an increasingly competitive environment because of planning and regulatory restrictions, changes in demand, and more aggressive behavior by other local health care providers. Community General Hospital is likely to be the major competitor because of its range of basic services, leading position in advanced medical technology, and aggressive behavior. Metropolitan Hospital and Lincoln County Hospital will compete in selected services. New health care providers are likely to compete with the hospital in areas of new opportunities, especially in outpatient care.

3. Basic beliefs

The following statements constitute the basic beliefs that will serve as the foundation and philosophical basis for the direction and operation of the hospital as it prepares for the future.

- General Hospital is a humanitarian organization designed to serve the health and medical needs of all members of society, particularly the citizens of northeast Lincoln County and, selectively, residents of communities in other parts of Lincoln County.
- The hospital should offer a broad range of basic medical services, plus selected specialty, health promotion, and disease prevention services for adults and children on both an inpatient and ambulatory basis.
- The quality of all of the hospital's services should exceed minimum mandated standards.
- The hospital offers professional education programs to enhance the quality of care and to increase the pool of skilled health professionals in the hospital and community.
- The hospital has a continuing commitment to the education of professional nurses in its school of nursing.
- The hospital operates free of discrimination of any kind.
- The hospital involves all affected parties in the hospital in a participative, consultative process of change.
- The hospital espouses a philosophy of dynamic conservatism that synchronizes the development of the hospital's plans, resources, and priorities with demonstrated community needs and other external forces.
- Private practices are supported as the primary model of medical care delivery; however, other forms of organization may be effective in specific situations.
- Cooperation with other local hospitals and agencies, including the possibility of participation in multi-institutional arrangements, is encouraged when it is consistent with the interests of this hospital.
- The hospital directs its own destiny and maintains its own identity. It will not be limited by location and existing relationships with other hospitals and agencies.

4. Strategy for markets and services
   The guidelines presented in this portion of the strategic plan relate to the services and markets to be considered by the hospital as it prepares for the future. General Hospital will seek to:
   - Sustain and, where appropriate, strengthen existing service and market positions, while expanding selectively and assertively into new markets, particularly in outpatient care
   - Develop a wide range of ambulatory services and secure an increasingly dominant market share
   - Improve the quality and scope of emergency services and secure an increasingly dominant share of this market
   - Establish a market position in geriatrics that incorporates an organized approach to the care of the aged, including a range of services from disease prevention through acute, extended, and terminal care
   - Develop a strong market position in health promotion and disease prevention that includes education, early diagnosis, screening, and preventive and behavior modification services
   - Increase the percentage share of the northeastern Lincoln County market and attract more patients from areas of the county by increasing physician awareness of hospital services, recruiting medical staff from outlying towns, and developing new services that will attract physicians and patients
   - Examine other opportunities (identified at the retreat): industrial medicine, dental care, extended care, hospital care, and rehabilitative care
5. Guidelines for competing
   To survive in an increasingly competitive environment, General Hospital must follow new guidelines for and relating to regulators and other health providers. Specifically, it must:
   - Behave more aggressively in relation to competing institutions and regulators
   - Develop strong positions in desired markets and services
   - Redress weaknesses on a selected basis, for example, CT scanners and linear accelerators
   - Sharpen its analysis of competitive institutions
   - Anticipate and respond to new developments in health and medicine and in the hospital environment
   - Pursue crucial regulatory approvals more aggressively
   - Execute approved plans rapidly
6. Guidelines for implementation
   As a means of fulfilling its destiny as defined in this strategic plan, General Hospital must develop new skills, attitudes, and resources. It must therefore:
   - Improve the effectiveness of the board of trustees by achieving greater diversity of membership, strengthening trustee education, examining the structure and workings of the board and its committees, and encouraging trustees to be more active and challenging
   - Develop medical staff leadership at all levels through better communication with and appropriate involvement of physicians in program planning and operations
   - Carry out organized recruitment of well-trained physician specialists, with particular emphasis on primary care physicians
   - Establish improved house coverage in all major clinical specialties by strengthening existing residency programs and house staff arrangements, while continuing to consider new residencies in primary specialties and a medical school affiliation
   - Develop in-house resources and capabilities, particularly in planning and marketing, to successfully operate the hospital in a rapidly changing, competitive environment
   - Maintain an adequate supply of well-trained employees, with particular emphasis on nursing, by offering competitive wage and benefits programs, effective continuing education, and a strong school of nursing
   - Establish an aggressive capital budgeting program to provide for continuing improvements of the hospital's physical facilities and equipment and for the resources required for new services

- Maintain the hospital's physical facilities by developing and implementing long-range plans for mechanical and energy management systems
- Enhance the hospital's image in the community by conducting a marketing study with professional assistance and by instituting required action to correct identified problems
- Secure new sources of funding and protect these funds by establishing a foundation and an in-house development capability
- Evaluate the effectiveness of the Intercity Hospital Fund and make whatever changes are appropriate
- Turn planning controls to the hospital's advantage through superior strategic planning, political influence, and an external affairs capability
- Investigate the feasibility of providing services in satellite locations and develop a position on participation in multi-institutional arrangements

Strategy and Corporate Governance

"The mastery of the concept of strategy makes easier the kind of discussion in boardrooms that help management make better decisions. It performs this function by reducing the world of detail to be considered to those central aspects of external environment and internal resources that affect the company and bear on the definition of its business. The special skill involved in perceiving and communicating the strategic significance of a business decision may be of the highest importance in engaging independent directors in the exercise of their assumed responsibility and in establishing active and effective boards as normal adjuncts to competent professional management."

—Kenneth R. Andrews, *The Concept of Corporate Strategy*[5]

Lourdes Hospital

Lourdes Hospital is a 320-bed, two-unit hospital that is owned and operated by a Catholic order of nuns. Both units serve suburban markets and are separated by approximately 12 miles. The two facilities are units of a single organization with common governance and management and many shared services. However, the medical staffs are distinct and different.

Much of the hospital's planning centered on program development and construction of the second facility. The hiring of an outside consultant to conduct a strategic planning retreat reflects management's awareness that something else was needed to guide the future activities of the institution. The following statement of strategy reflects the findings and deliberations of the Strategic Planning Committee at a 1-1/2 day retreat conducted in a hotel in December 1981. It is based on the belief that Lourdes Hospital must develop general directions and guidelines for the future as essential first steps in carrying out its strategic planning efforts. These findings will be applied and adapted, as may be required, to both of the units (North and South) operated by the hospital.

The statement of strategy is organized into the following major sections:

1. Introduction
2. Conclusions from environmental analysis
3. Triggers for change: emerging opportunities and challenges
4. Basic beliefs
5. A basic challenge for the future
6. General guidelines for future strategies
7. Basic directions and opportunities

1. Introduction

As a community-oriented health services institution, Lourdes Hospital must be alert to what is taking place in the outside environment in which it operates and to the changing needs and expectations of the population that it intends to serve. From time to time—and this is a propitious time—Lourdes Hospital must evaluate its resources and operations in terms of the ability to adapt to new conditions. The hospital must be prepared to adopt new strategies in order to meet new challenges and opportunities and minimize or avert new threats to its future development.

A statement of strategy provides a framework for choices about the direction Lourdes Hospital intends to follow in adjusting to changing conditions in the outside world and the specific requirements of its local health care market. In making these choices, the hospital will be guided by the basic beliefs that form the basis of its work as a Catholic general hospital and as a community health service institution. These beliefs offer both opportunities for future service and limitations on the type and scope of services that the hospital intends to provide.

This statement is also intended to shape the future planning efforts that will be carried out by the recently formed Strategic Planning Committee. In this sense, this statement is simply an underpinning for the future development and operation of Lourdes Hospital as it prepares for the world of tomorrow.

2. Conclusions from environmental analysis

Religious forces

- The decline in vocations to the sponsoring order and a concurrent drop in interest in institutional service by postulants and sisters must be recognized. This will result in more lay involvement in the management of Lourdes Hospital. However, there is little the hospital, as an institution, can do to reverse this trend.
- Certain basic moral beliefs about abortion, euthanasia, and other matters that affect the dignity of the individual must be taken into consideration in planning new services. At times, general public sentiments and expectations may conflict with the basic religious beliefs of the hospital's apostolate. The hospital must be prepared to address these issues, fully recognizing that very difficult decisions may be involved, particularly in a pluralistic society where everyone may not share its beliefs.

Technological advances

- The great advances that have taken place in medical technology will continue to make heavy demands on all hospitals. Advances in genetic engineering, breakthroughs in cancer therapy, and reduced need for exploratory surgery are just three developments that promise to affect the scope and types of services in the future.
- The hospital must carefully monitor these advances and be prepared to adopt whatever new technology is needed to accomplish its long-term goals and that is appropriate to its resource capabilities.

Economic forces

- The steady increase in hospital costs in recent decades has generated much public concern and government intervention. Although some changes may occur in regulatory mechanisms, stringent restrictions are expected to continue. These restrictions will reduce length of stay, inpatient admissions, and use of hospital services and will encourage the use of less expensive alternatives to inpatient care. The hospital must be prepared to adjust to these changes through increased productivity, careful containment of costs, and utilization review programs.
- Hospitals will continue to seek outside capital, mainly through money markets, to finance new construction and new programs. The competition for such funds promises to increase. The hospital is fortunate that it will not need to seek additional funds for these purposes in the near future.

Demographic trends

- Several demographic realities and trends will have an impact on the work of all hospitals. The number of persons aged 65 and older is projected to increase from approximately 25 million, or 11 percent of the U.S. population in 1980, to approximately 55 million, or slightly more than 18 percent, in 2030. Increases in the average life span and improvements in the overall health of the aged may reduce the need for health and hospital services, but may raise new problems and issues that cannot be foreseen. The quality of life and related matters, such as euthanasia, will emerge as public issues. The hospital must be prepared to deal with these issues when they arise.

- The decline in the national birth rate will result in a decrease in demand in neonatal and obstetric services. However, there are indications that this trend may not pertain to the population served by this hospital.
- The nation is experiencing considerable internal migration, primarily through the flight of populations from central cities to suburbs and from frostbelt to sunbelt states. These changes are also taking place in the local markets served by the two units of Lourdes Hospital. The 1980 census shows that virtually all of Jackson County's growth in the previous decade was in the three southern townships. Continued high growth is projected in these townships. Hospitals serving these markets should be alert to increased demands for health and hospital services resulting from this growth in population.

Social and political changes

- Recent Medicaid and other federal cutbacks may result in a return to local responsibility for the financing and provision of health care services to the poor. This could place heavy burdens on institutions that have an historic commitment to providing care to the disadvantaged and poor.
- A growing disillusionment in the ability of the federal government to address social and economic problems has resulted in major political shifts and in a return to local solutions. More important, funding of such solutions may shift to the local level. This shift makes it even more imperative that the hospital develop the capability to survive with less government assistance. The adoption of new policies and practices that emphasize economic survival over community service may be required.

Developments and trends in the health care industry

- In the next decade, a significant increase in the number of physicians and other health care practitioners (except, perhaps, registered nurses) is expected. In this same period, nurses and other medical practitioners will demand greater authority in the practice of their professions in hospitals. As these essential clinical practitioners compete for authority and for use of hospital resources, hospitals must address these issues to the satisfaction of all concerned. Lourdes Hospital must be prepared to review its present practices and policies on medical staff appointments, credentialing, and the employment of nurses and other health care professionals as an essential first step in creating a more attractive environment for the practice of these professions and in encouraging greater staff involvement in the affairs of the institution.
- The hospital industry is consolidating, and the number and types of multi-institutional arrangements are expected to increase. With few exceptions, efforts toward the development of such arrangements have lagged in this part of the state. There are strong possibilities that such arrangements, particularly in the form of satellite and outreach facilities, will increase. The hospital must be alert to these developments, both in terms of new opportunities and emerging threats to its own programs.
- There has been a striking increase in the number of investor-owned hospitals nationwide. To date, this development has not taken place in this state, although it is perhaps only a matter of time when investor-owned chains will penetrate this market. This hospital and other voluntary institutions must be prepared to meet this challenge by adopting more aggressive marketing efforts, adding needed services, and emphasizing cooperative arrangements.
- Increasing emphasis on wellness programs and preventive medicine has encouraged many hospitals to develop programs in these areas. Although several local hospitals have already established such activities, at times with limited success, ample opportunities exist for new and imaginative services. These programs are a natural extension of this hospital's traditional concern for meeting the total health needs of its patients and its local community.
- The demand for collective bargaining and the resulting unionization of hospital employees continues to grow. Some of the local inner city hospitals have been involved in recent efforts. This hospital should be prepared to deal with the matter in a forthright

manner by ensuring that its personnel policies and practices, working conditions, salaries, fringe benefits, opportunities for advancement and participation, and other inducements meet or exceed local community norms and expectations. As a Catholic institution, the hospital is fortunate that it can refer to recent papal encyclicals on this important subject.

- At the national level, a thrust exists to reduce health care regulation, especially restrictions on entry into the market. However, it is not possible at this time to determine how this may affect certificate-of-need and other health regulatory programs in this state. Should certificate-of-need regulation diminish or disappear entirely in the state, considerable activity in the establishment of new programs and services, creation of new facilities, and market penetration by investor-owned chains can be expected. The hospital must be prepared to adopt new strategies that will enable it to defend its present market position or improve its market share to avert the threats of new competition.

3. Triggers for change: emerging opportunities and challenges
   After considerable discussion, the following opportunities and challenges in the environment were identified as areas that might greatly affect the future of the hospital and its service programs:
   - The return to local responsibility for care of the poor and accompanying economic constraints
   - Problems of caring for patients 65 and older, particularly in the market served by the South unit
   - Potential decline in demand for pediatric services at the North unit
   - Emerging physician surplus and nurse shortage and the problems associated with solving these manpower problems
   - The threat of increased competition, particularly from investor-owned hospitals
   - Increased emphasis and concurrent opportunities for wellness and related preventive health care services
   - New opportunities to strengthen and broaden multi-institutional arrangements
   - The need to keep abreast of rapid developments in medical technology and to replace obsolete, expensive high technology
4. Basic Beliefs
   The following statements constitute the beliefs that serve as the foundation and philosophical basis for the direction and operation of Lourdes Hospital as it prepares for the future:
   - The Catholic tradition makes the hospital different from other local community hospitals. Its mission and programs cannot be separated from the overall mission and philosophy of the Sisters of St. Gregory the Great. This tradition and philosophy forms the basis of all that the hospital at present does or aspires to do.
   - The work of the hospital is guided by a belief in the dignity of each person who seeks its services or who works within its walls, and by a respect for the needs and values of all persons with whom it comes into contact. It aspires to provide its services in a compassionate manner, with an emphasis on hospitality, courtesy, and personalized care. In keeping with this philosophy, within the resource capabilities of the institution, no patient will be denied care who requires it. Patients who require a service not available at either unit will be referred to other local institutions where such care is available.
   - The hospital recognizes that it must attract sufficient resources to enable it to carry out its service obligations and to meet unexpected contingencies. Therefore, its revenues must exceed its expenses so that interest and loan payments can be promptly met and so that funds will be available to establish new services and replace equipment, as needed.
   - The hospital aspires to provide an array of programs and services capable of meeting the health care needs of its local community and to provide these services in an economical manner, stressing a quality of care that exceeds generally accepted national standards. However, it will carefully examine all requests for highly sophisticated tertiary services that require expensive equipment and highly trained personnel and for which a sufficient market or demand may not exist to underwrite these services.
   - The hospital's financial plans and capital financing activities are based on the belief that

acquiring capital through borrowing is legitimate and prudent and that the provision for interest payments and reduction of principal is a justifiable patient care expense.

- The hospital realizes that it must carefully control costs and avoid waste. Specifically, its financial management is based on the premise that a sound budgeting process must control expenditures.
- In providing hospital and related health care services, the hospital recognizes that these must be readily acceptable and accessible to the patients it intends to serve. Wherever feasible, the hospital will provide these services in convenient locations and in environments that are safe and pleasant. This belief has already led to the creation and continuing modernization of its two local facilities.
- The hospital strives to keep abreast of changes in medical education, technology, new practices, and knowledge through the establishment of new programs, acquisition of new equipment, changes in medical practice, and a continuing emphasis on planning.
- The hospital will cooperate with other local hospitals and agencies, including the possibility of further participation in multi-institutional arrangements when the activities are consistent with its interests.
- The hospital will continue to be guided by the philosophy that basic health care services are best delivered and received in the local community. Therefore, the hospital must maintain its identity and direct its affairs with the best interests of its community always in mind.

5. A basic challenge for the future

Lourdes Hospital has accomplished much in developing a local Catholic health care system through the organization and construction of its South unit in 1979. Although the two facilities are units of a common organizational structure with single governance and management and with shared services in all major departments, two distinct and different medical staffs exist. To date, referrals between the two institutions have been limited. In part, this is the result of the different geographic orientation of the physicians at the two institutions. The medical staff of the South unit is younger, oriented more toward inner city hospitals. Because of the newness of the South unit, its medical staff has not had time to develop as strong a commitment to the institution as have the physicians at the North unit.

There are limited exchanges of courtesy privileges between the two units, but no sharing of medical education activities. These factors also discourage referrals between the two units, and many patients are referred to competitor institutions for services not currently available at one of the facilities.

To ensure the survival of both institutions in an increasingly competitive environment, it may be necessary to explore new arrangements for greater cooperation and increased referrals by physicians at the two institutions. This is perhaps the most pressing challenge facing the development of a unified Lourdes health care system.

6. General guidelines for future strategies

As a means of fulfilling its destiny as described in this statement, Lourdes Hospital must develop new skills, attitudes, and resources based on the following guidelines.

Competition

- In its effort to survive in an increasingly competitive environment, the hospital will not violate its basic philosophy and values as a Christian humanitarian health care institution. This is not to imply, however, that the hospital will not behave more aggressively in relation to competing institutions and regulators, as future conditions may dictate.
- The hospital will develop strong positions in desired markets and services. It will not compete in "losers," except where there are important unmet community needs such as when the life and safety of patients in its local market are at stake.
- The hospital will not consider the introduction of services that violate Christian ethics and the philosophy of the Sisters of St. Gregory the Great.
- The hospital will compete by introducing new technology and new services that will

enable it to do what it is at present doing but in a more effective, more efficient, or more productive manner. It will consider the introduction of new services to meet unmet or emerging community health needs, provided that it can muster the necessary resource and know-how to manage these services. In this respect, the hospital sees no need at this time to compete by developing services that already exist and are adequately performed in its local market.

Growth and opportunities

- The hospital will anticipate and respond to new developments in health, medicine, and hospital care.
- The hospital will consider establishing new tertiary and other sophisticated services only if it can mobilize the necessary resources and justify their efficient use and if the services are not available at distances convenient to its patients.
- The hospital considers growth an asset *only* when such growth meets local community needs, is compatible with the institution's basic philosophies and mission, is economically feasible, and when it can be managed efficiently.

Diversification

- In accordance with the above provisos, the hospital is prepared to consider the addition of new services and programs that it does not presently provide. Such activities can include any appropriate services ranging from traditional medical and hospital programs to new, unrelated income-producing ventures.
- The hospital will be alert to opportunities to expand its capabilities and influence, for example, outreach services, satellite operations, and medical office buildings, that generate additional revenues, enhance its community image and political influence, and attract new business, provided that these opportunities do not violate its basic mission and beliefs.
- The hospital will not, however, consider engaging in any activity for which a strong and steady demand does not exist or for which it cannot develop the management capabilities.

Cost containment strategy

- The hospital will strive to remain a low-cost producer by carrying out aggressive cost containment strategies and promoting increased productivity.
- These are essential steps in competing in the local health care market and in meeting community expectation for low health care costs.

Corporate restructuring

- The hospital will carefully review opportunities to reorganize its corporate structure.
- These activities will enable the hospital to capitalize on new opportunities for diversification, provide new products and services, protect its assets, or meet local community needs more efficiently.

Sharing and multi-institutional arrangements

- The hospital will encourage and promote the continued exploration of opportunities for joint planning with St. John's Hospital and Our Lady of Patoma Hospital.
- The hospital will also participate in any multi-institutional sharing ventures that will enhance its ability to provide existing or new services in a more effective and efficient manner.

7. Basic directions and opportunities

The following is a list of opportunities and challenges that will be brought to the attention of the Strategic Planning Committee for its consideration and recommendations:

- Increase and strengthen the referral patterns between the hospital's two units
- Identify and assess local community expectations, attitudes, and perceptions toward the hospital and its work, and take corrective measures to improve the hospital's image
- Expand the hospital's market through establishment of outreach programs, including new satellite operations
- Consider opportunities for diversifying its activities
- Provide wellness and related health education services

- Encourage new religious (ecumenical) ventures that expand the hospital's commitment to a broader Judeo-Christian ministry and, more specifically, strengthen its pastoral care programs
- Translate its basic values into day-to-day operating procedures, recognizing emerging challenges to the hospital's basic mission and philosophy
- Evaluate its efforts, programs, and activities, employing evaluative norms and criteria of the Catholic Health Care Association

Four Characteristics of Good Strategy Statements

"1. They should describe each of the major components of the organization's strategy (that is, its scope, its resource deployments and distinctive competencies, its competitive advantages and how they will be produced, and its intended synergy).
2. They should indicate how the strategy will lead to the accomplishment of the organization's objectives.
3. The strategy should be described in functional, rather than physical, terms.
4. The strategy statement should be as precise as possible."

—Charles W. Hofer and Dan Schendel, *Strategy Formulation: Analytical Concepts*[6]

Analysis of Strategic Plans

The following questions are helpful in analyzing strategic plans such as the two presented in this chapter:

- Do the two strategy statements provide a clear sense of direction for the institutions' future efforts?
- Do the statements indicate that the preparers of the strategies were aware of outside threats and opportunities and their potential impact on the work of the institutions?
- Do these strategies appear to reflect (1) the personal values and aspirations of top management, (2) shared corporate values of the organization as a whole, and (3) desired organizational commitments to society?
- Will the strategies help the hospitals' leaders decide on future programs and services and the clientele to be served?
- Will they be useful in priority decisions for acquiring new equipment and in allocating staff, space, and financial resources?
- Will the strategies be easy to communicate to others?
- Are the strategies reasonable and workable? Are they perhaps too comprehensive? Do they attempt to do too much? If so, how would you alter them?
- Will these strategies enable the managements of these hospitals to deal with existing or new competitors in what may be a more competitive future environment?
- Is your hospital ready to carry out a similar effort and develop a written strategy patterned on these strategies? Do you believe that your hospital's assessments and responses will differ substantially from those presented in the two examples?

Three Corporate Strategies Summarized

"Ingersoll-Rand has continued to grow in this changing world. Diversification is a key element in that success. We are diversified in the wide range of products we manufacture, in the variety and breadth of our markets, and in the worldwide scope of our operations."

—Ingersoll-Rand Co., 1980 Annual Report

"Tg's strategy for growth and profitability remains the same . . . [Tg] continues to grow in natural resources and related businesses with operations favorably positioned, primarily in North America. We intend to remain a low-cost producer and to concentrate on products for which demand is strong and growing."

—Richard D. Mollison, chairman of the board, Texasgulf, Inc., 1980 Annual Report

"As part of the company's ongoing strategic approach to improving returns, we've been taking three specific types of action:

- We are making certain that we support fully those businesses in which Olin has a strong competitive position. . . .
- For the remaining businesses, as objectively as possible, we are determining what is required in terms of additional resources, money, and key people to achieve a leadership position.
- Once we have made a decision on the future potential of a business for us, we will either commit the additional resources or, on a planned basis, exit from the business."

—Olin Corporation, 1980 Annual Report

Notes

1. Abell, Derek F. *Defining The Business: The Starting Point of Strategic Planning.* Englewood Cliffs, NJ: Prentice-Hall, Inc., 1980, p. 218.

2. Campbell, Ph.D., David. *If You Don't Know Where You're Going, You'll Probably End up Somewhere Else.* Niles, IL: Argus Communications, 1974, p. 102.

3. Rothschild, William E. *Putting It All Together: A Guide to Strategic Thinking.* New York City: AMACOM, 1976.

4. Andrews, Kenneth R. *The Concept of Corporate Strategy.* 1980 revised edition. Homewood, IL: Richard D. Irwin, Inc., 1980, p. 85.

5. Andrews, p. 85.

6. Hofer, Charles W., and Schendel, Dan. *Strategy Formulation: Analytical Concepts.* St. Paul: West Publishing Company, 1978, p. 42.

Chapter 11

From Strategic Thinking to Strategic Management

"If strategy deals with the long term, the precedent setting, and the commitment of critical resources, then the process of developing strategy is the nonroutine activity of altering normal patterns of planning and operations."

—Joseph L. Bower and Yves Doz, *Strategic Management: A New View of Business Policy and Planning*[1]

"Strategic leadership has been a rare phenomenon in the nonprofits. On infrequent occasions, a visionary and charismatic individual sets out to lead his university, or hospital, to a position of prominence. . . . Typically, creative leadership occurs during the early days of a nonprofit. As it grows and matures it settles into the typical stable pattern, where strategic change is minimal, local, occasional, unguided, caused by external stimuli."

—H. Igor Ansoff, *Strategic Management*[2]

"To be caught utterly unprepared for opportunities that are possible and foreseeable, even if unlikely, is among the worst forms of a generalship that takes counsel of its fears."

—Russell F. Weigley, *Eisenhower's Lieutenants: The Campaigns of France and Germany 1944-1945*[3]

"[L]ife is somewhat like when you're on a boat and there is a wind blowing. You can't control the wind, but if you set your sails right, you can get to your destination."

—William Hornady, Ph.D., *Modern Maturity*[4]

Although a distinction is often made between the management of day-to-day operations and the management of change, executives in many types of enterprises increasingly recognize that the two tasks are inextricably interwoven into a new way of managing known as *strategic management.* Not only must managers look inward at the workings of their organizations (the traditional concern of management), but also they must be continually alert to what is happening in the outside environment and how this may affect internal operations (the outside-in approach). Perceptive managers now realize that getting the job done efficiently is no longer enough; they must learn to manage change, as well.[5]

This book has thus far concerned itself with strategic thinking, dividing the process into two major components, *analysis and diagnosis* and *strategy formulation.* However, it has recognized that two subsequent actions, *linking the resulting strategy with the planning process* and *integrating the strategy into the overall management of the organization,* are equally important. This concluding chapter discusses these two subsequent actions, much of which is new to hospitals. It is new in the sense that many hospital authorities do not think in these terms, although many of their decisions reflect an instinctive awareness of the impact of outside forces on management policies and decisions.

The key point of this chapter, how strategy meshes with the overall planning and management of an organization, is introduced best with a recapitulation of the basic concepts of strategic thinking. Strategy is a focused concept for the development and operation of an organization (see chapter 1). It suggests that a hospital can muster resources to its advantage, determine the market or clientele it expects to serve, and develop new services within its resource capabilities and within existing regulatory guidelines to meet the needs of its clientele or market. It provides a framework to guide the choices that determine how a hospital interacts with a changing world. It supplies both direction and cohesion to the institution. *Strategy implies, above all, that the institution can make certain choices that enable it to effectively match its internal capabilities and managerial competencies with the changing demands and opportunities of its outside world. In short, it allows hospital management to optimize the fit between the institution and the environment.*

Responses to Environmental Forces

"Responses to environmental forces are fundamentally of two types—either modify the forces or make strategy changes, or use some combination of both. Attempts to modify forces are often unsuccessful, and such attempts may be impossible. . . . The more common response is for the organization to alter its strategies to reduce the potential impact of the environmental force on the firm."

—D. W. Cravens and others,
Marketing Decision Making: Concepts and Strategy[6]

These choices often result in some sections of the market getting more and other sections getting fewer services. This, in turn, leads to an accompanying asymmetry in allocation of resources, funds, and staff within an organization's departments and programs. This notion of asymmetry—the unequal treatment and allocation of resources and services by an organization—is a pervasive element of strategy. Rarely is an organization in a position to allocate its resources and services equally among competing demands. Most managers learn to work within these restrictions, albeit not always comfortably.

Because of their role as environment-serving organizations,[7] hospitals increasingly find themselves in new situations that limit their abilities or desires to provide a comprehensive array of high-quality, multilevel diagnostic, preventive, curative, and restorative health care services to everyone who may need these services. Balancing a goal of being all things to all people with available and potential resources is a matter of strategy, a matter of adjusting what the institution would like to do with what its resources will allow it to do. These choices are difficult to make and, therefore, are best made within the framework of an overall institutional strategy.

Hospitals do not always consciously make these tough choices; outside forces often impose these choices upon them. A question that regularly stimulates heated discussion at strategic retreats is, "Would you summarize your hospital's actions as the result of its *ambitions* or a reaction to outside conditions?'' The usual response is that the hospital arose originally from the ambitions of its founders to meet a specific need or capitalize on a new opportunity. In time, changing conditions may have forced many actions that no longer reflect these original ambitions or purposes. For example, despite a hospital's ambition to serve everyone in need of its services, inadequate reimbursement or dwindling endowments may now require it to limit elective admissions to patients who are able to pay directly for their care or who are covered by various third-party arrangements. Changing times, local competition, medical staff demands, or accreditation requirements, rather than the ambitions of the hospital's leaders, may also trigger the introduction of new technology, the acquisition of specialized equipment, the organization of new programs, or the imposition of higher standards. Of course, the question posed at retreats is deliberately tantalizing to arouse discussion. Most hospitals are the products of both ambition and condition. Strategic thinking is simply a disciplined way of determining which is the appropriate response at the moment, thereby ensuring a continuing fit between the institution and its environment.

Strategy also implies that there is usually a best time to act, that there is a period of time during which a ''strategic window'' is open to allow an organization to capitalize on outside opportunities. Harassed as most managers seem to be by pressing day-to-day operating problems, it is understandable that so few of them recognize the importance of anticipating the future before it looms up on them as the present. By then, it may be too late for effective action, because the strategic window is no longer open. Managers must change their basic management styles to reflect the new realities of a rapidly changing, turbulent environment. They must move away from an introspective approach that focuses on internal activities to an outside-in management style that forces them to be more sensitive to external change; this shift will better prepare them to cope with change.

Strategic Window

''Timing is an important element in strategic management. Indeed, ''there are often only limited periods when the 'fit' between the 'key requirements' of a market and the particular competences of a firm competing in that market are at an optimum. Investment in a product line or market area has to be timed to coincide with periods in which a *strategic window* is open, that is, where a close fit exists. Disinvestment should be considered if, during the course of the market's evolution, changes in market requirements outstrip the firm's capability to adapt itself to the new circumstances.

''The strategic window concept can be useful to incumbent competitors as well as to would-be entrants into a market. For the former it provides a way of relating future strategic moves to market evolution and of assessing how resources should be allocated to existing activities. For the latter it provided a framework for diversification and new entry.''

—Derek F. Abell and John S. Hammond, *Strategic Market Planning: Problems and Analytical Approaches*[8]

In addition, strategic thinking imposes a rationality on the management process. It encourages managers to think in terms of present and future trends, emerging issues, and new opportunities and threats and to devise effective ways for the organization to deal with them. A good strategy presupposes that the decision maker will select the option best suited to achieve desired ends by thoughtful analysis of available information, reasonable conclusions, and appropriate actions, and not by off-the-cuff remarks, emotional choices, or chance selection. Indeed, a major contribution of strategic thinking to good management is the rationality that it imposes on the organization's efforts to anticipate and control its future.

A striking development during the past two decades has been the growing acceptance of long-range planning as an essential ingredient of hospital management. Planning is not new to the health care scene; hospitals and other health service organizations have traditionally carried out some form of planning whenever they constructed new facilities, established new programs, or expanded existing services. In recent years, planning has been promoted as an essential condition for hospital survival and as a means of containing rising health care costs. Both the literature and government actions have reflected this new emphasis.[9]

Much planning performed by hospitals can be described as *operational planning*. This is basically a bottom-up, cyclical (iterative), internally focused process involving top management and department heads. It is closely allied to the preparation of annual operating budgets, three-year capital expenditure plans, and human resources planning. This type of planning is promoted by section 234 of P.L. 92-603 and by the Joint Commission on Accreditation of Hospitals. It is essential to good management, but something else is needed for an institution to deal with the uncontrollable, uncertain futures. This something else, of course, is strategy.

Many managers continue to confuse strategy with planning. Some commit the more serious error of divorcing both from daily operations. Others move too quickly into operational planning without making the strategic decisions that should precede and support planning. Or, they fail to convert their planning decisions into future operations, seemingly trusting that once a plan is put on paper, it will magically produce results.[10] Typically, many managers breathe a sigh of relief when the planning task is completed; they can now return to the real business of running the organization. Even more disastrous, some managers fail to realize that managing in terms of long-range goals—the objectives-first approach—no longer may be valid in a turbulent environment, in a climate where so many outside groups are telling hospitals what and what not to do, or in situations where resources are in scarce supply.[11]

Strategic management, *an integrative process that links strategic thinking with the overall planning and management of an enterprise,* is a new way of managing. It is more than simply expanding previous notions of planning and management. It rests on several key approaches:

- *Distinguishing* between strategy and operations, between the formulation of the strategy and implementing it, and between strategic thinking and short-term or long-term operational planning
- Adopting a *programmatic perspective* that recognizes the interplay among the various organizational units and programs that constitute the structural elements of an institution[12]
- Recognizing the *levels of control* that underlie the management and coordination of these structual elements
- Emphasizing *future uncertainty* and its implications in managerial decision making

Most of these concepts have already been discussed in this book because they are fundamental to the strategic thinking process. However, some additional words are necessary to describe how strategic management fits into the overall managerial framework of an institution. Again, it must be emphasized that strategic management, like strategy, is a line management effort; indeed, it can only be done by top management, although staff can contribute to the process. It involves the entire workings of the organization and links all the programs and elements into a meaningful operating entity. It starts with the proposition that the organization exists *because* of its environment, that the environment is the starting point for all planning and managerial decisions. Finally, strategic management is future-oriented and focuses on ways of managing change in an increasingly uncertain future environment (see figure 13, The Basic Elements and Relationships in Strategic Planning and Management).

Strategic management is an approach to managing a complex enterprise in a world of change. It is neither easy to do nor easy to learn. There are so many operating demands on a manager's time that a determined commitment is essential to carrying out the notion. Moreover, managers must also be patient because considerable time is required to devise or evolve a satisfactory strategic management process. Indeed, it can at times be rather messy and loose. There is very little tried and proven advice that can be offered in encouraging this new style of management, except to state that it requires continual learning and experience to make it work successfully.[13]

Strategic management is based on a premise that, once expressed, is quite simple: *environmental change also demands changes in the overall strategy and structure of the enterprise itself.* Strategy and structure are familiar to management theorists, and much of the strategic management literature in the past has emphasized strategy formulation and the resulting restructuring of organizations.[15] But a new framework has recently been introduced by Thomas J. Peters. This framework recognizes that the strategy-structure model is insufficient to explain what really takes place in complex organizations. Therefore, Peters specifies seven variables: *structure, strategy, systems, skills, staff, style,* and

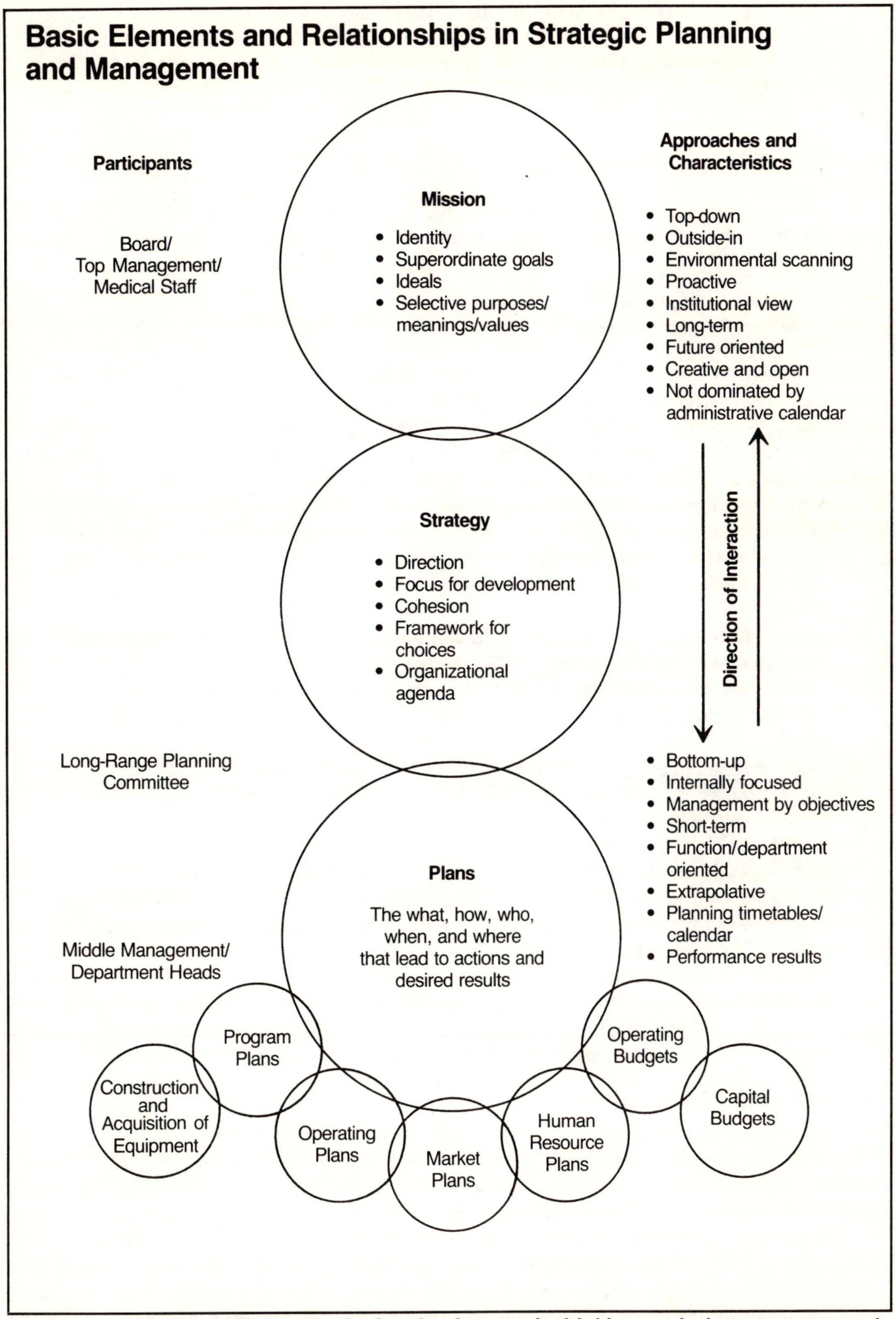

Figure 13. This figure illustrates the levels of strategic thinking—mission, strategy, and plans—their relationship with one another, and the interaction among the numerous approaches and characteristics.

Use What You Have to Decide What You Want to Do

"What could be rationally wrong with collectively considering where we want to go and what might be the best way of getting there? So much is wrong it is hard to know where to begin. The question itself is confusing. Does destination know no limitation? Do we first decide where and then how? The priority is perverse; it is no better than the reverse, as if the journey always mattered more than the destination. No, where one wishes to go depends on whether one is able to get there. Life is larger than our categories. When my grandfather lost the family fortune comprised of fifty rubles, he went to see the local miracle rabbi, Joseph of Slutsk, who consulted mystical works, and told him to collect ten kopecks apiece from his friends and relatives and take it to the train. 'But where shall I go?' Grandpa cited. 'As far as your money will take you,' replied the rabbi, who knew more about the relationship of resources to objectives than his seemingly scientific successors."

—Aaron Wildavsky, *Speaking Truth to Power: The Art and Craft of Policy Analysis*[14]

superordinate goals. All seven are equally important. When dealing with change, an organization must take all seven into account, both as a change program checklist and as a means of collecting information to diagnose problems associated with change. Peters terms the last five the "soft 5," because they are purported to be the softest ones, the ones that involve people and what they do and believe in. However, these are always the hardest to change; hence his claim "soft is hard."[16]

- *Structure* embraces not only the way in which an enterprise is organized (its organizational design, departmentalization, and degree of centralization), but also its internal hierarchies and roles and interrelationships of the various units and program elements. It is the muscle and vital organs of an organization and is usually depicted as an organizational chart.
- *Strategy* is the framework for making the choices that determine how the institution will interact with a changing world.
- *Systems* are the language of an enterprise, what makes it click and work as an entity. Examples include the budget system, promotion system, reward system, and formal planning system.
- *Skills* refer to distinctive collective capabilities exhibited by the organization as a whole rather than skills of the persons within the organization. They are the things that the organization does well or poorly and that characterize its efforts.
- *Staff* is the human dimension, with all that this implies in terms of human relations, staffing, performance, training, competence, morale, and job security.
- *Style* is a two-fold variable. One aspect concerns management style: how managers behave, how they spend their time, and how much hands-on attention they give to key themes. The other aspect relates to the style of the business as a whole: its culture and orientation and how it carries out its business.
- *Superordinate* goals are the shared values and beliefs that bind the fabric of an organization. They are, in a sense, the reason people come to work. As Peters observes, "They're short, sloganlike, frequently not meaningful at first, particularly to outsiders. . . . "Almost all of these could be considered 'motherhoods' . . . [that] over a period of years have taken on great meaning in each institution."[17] These are what usually drive strategy. More important, they clearly delineate what is strategically out of bounds.

The notion of superordinate goals is akin to the concept of organizational mission. In chapter 2, a mission statement was described as being either the jumping-off point for the formulation of strategy or one of the outcomes of the strategic management process. For hospitals wrestling with questions of basic values, such as the appropriate balance between social responsibility and economic performance, the explicit consideration of mission separate from strategy may be desirable. Mission in this context refers to philosophy, aspirations, ideals, and purpose: what the hospital stands for, whether it emphasizes profits and growth, community service, or the healing ministry. A productive way to formulate this type of mission statement is by using a portion of the idealized design approach advocated by Russell Ackoff (see Idealized Design Approach).

Idealized Design Approach

The idealized design approach is a way of formulating a mission that combines analytical and systems thinking to design an ideal future and invent ways to bring it about. An ideal is a long-term goal that is believed to be unattainable, but toward which progress is possible during and after the period planned for. It is particularly useful under conditions of uncertainty where predict-and-prepare approaches fall short. It helps institutions to overcome self-imposed constraints and to articulate what they really stand for.

Step 1: Developing a reference scenario
- What is our current status and direction?
- What ends are espoused by the organization but are not actually pursued? What internal conflicts are holding us back?
- If we were to project our basic indicators for the next five years, what would they look like?
- Given the answers to these questions, what is the most likely scenario for our institution if there were no significant changes in its behavior and in its environment?

Step 2: Develop an ideal redesign
- What would we like to see as the mission, selective purpose, or superordinate goal of the organization?
- Ideally, what characteristics should the organization possess (in terms of role, markets, services, competition, performance, organization, staff, and relationships with external bodies)?
- What should be done to endow the organization with the desired characteristics?

Step 3: Comparison of reference with ideal
- What gaps are apparent between our reference scenario and our idealized design?

Step 4: Inventing ways to fill the gaps
- What are the means for filling these gaps?

When applying this approach in a strategic retreat, the first step usually results in a dissatisfaction with continuing as is; this, in turn, creates an impetus to define a more desirable state, the ideal. The idealized design becomes a statement of heartfelt aspirations that, in fact, leads to a statement of mission.

—Adapted from Russell L. Ackoff,
Creating the Corporate Future,
copyright © 1981 by
John Wiley & Sons[18]

The seven variables cited provide simple but powerful insights into what enables an organization to survive and succeed through time. The seven Ss are not likely to surprise anyone; they are familiar to managers at least in concept, if not in their precise wording. However, most managers are not accustomed to think of the *fit* among these seven crucial elements. Strategic success comes from recognizing and controlling this fit or, at least, preventing any misfit among the seven variables. Peters warns that "one variable out of whack can torpedo the best laid strategic plans."[19]

Managing change in a complex organization such as a hospital is essentially a hands-on task involving "an array of small steps, constant monitoring, and subsequent adjustment," which emerge from an "in-depth understanding (in seven S terms) of the cause of current and past, sensible at the time, behavior."[20] Unfortunately, many managers fail to recognize that as situations change, an organization may not be able to maintain its internal consistency any longer. Its structure no longer fits the situation nor is the organization able to maintain the necessary match with its environment. The organization now has two choices: it can continue to adapt to its environment by steadily redesigning its structure as needed, or it can hold on to its present structure until the fit with its environment becomes so bad that it is forced to change its internal configuration. Henry Mintzberg, a well-known authority on the subject, noted that "the choice is between evolution and revolution, between perpetual mild adaptation, which favors external fit over time, and infrequent major realignment, which favors internal consistency over time."[21]

Hospitals have traditionally pursued the latter strategy. Some hospitals have weakened and then died because they were unable to restructure themselves to conform to external change, a fate which happened to many specialty hospitals in the past. But this, too, is changing. Hospitals are now increasingly exploring corporate restructuring, multi-institutional arrangements, diversification, and other organizational options as major strategies for the future.

It should be evident by now that because of the nature of their organizational structure and historic traditions hospitals are not easily changed. Innovation is difficult for them, and many internal barriers must be overcome before they can interact effectively with a changing environment. Most of the time all that is possible is to heed T. J. Peters' advice to "get the *herd* heading roughly East or roughly West." Translated, this colorful analogy implies that hospital management usually cannot fine-tune internal responses to external stimuli; at best, all it can hope to accomplish is to do well enough, but not necessarily as well as possible.

What is the role of the hospital CEO in all of this? As the architect of purpose (see chapter 2) and a shaper of institutional values, the CEO determines and reinforces on a daily basis the superordinate goals, selective purposes, beliefs, and mission of the organization. As the chief strategist, he works with the 12 best thinkers and other persons in the organization in formulating a focus for development, establishing a framework for program choice, and maintaining a defensible competitive position, all of which provide direction and cohesion to the hospital.

Most CEOs continue to focus their attentions on operational planning, emphasizing such matters as capital and expense budgets, recruitment plans, and facilities development. However, many of them are recognizing that they must also pay attention to more basic tasks. They are learning to deal with change, either by carrying out the strategic thinking process described in this book, by installing and managing a formal planning system, or by relying on a series of ad hoc planning decisions made in response to issues and events as they arise.

Some Key Thoughts on Strategic Thinking

"As an organization grows, the difficulty in maintaining a strategic perspective increases. It becomes too large for the CEO to know all he needs to know. And yet, as an organization grows, strategic thinking capability becomes essential as a means of continuing survival and growth.

"The key to effective strategic thinking is knowing enough to outwit the competition.

"Many useful techniques are available to help the process along. But don't rely on them too much; they are simply means, not ends.

"Good strategic thinking is hard work and takes time. The key difference between a good strategy and a bad one often is the degree of insight or creativity that is brought to it.

"Explicitly forcing new ways of looking at a problem is a good way to test whether insight/creativity is there or not."
—Allan Kennedy, speech[22]

By now it should be clear to the reader that the latter two approaches are inadequate, that neither enables an institution to manage change in a turbulent environment. Today's CEOs must learn not only to think in strategic terms, but also to engage others in the institution to think in similar terms. They must also be willing to relinquish some personal power and control of information and become less irreplaceable. In so doing, CEOs are shaping their institutions' capacity to respond to outside events in a more timely and effective manner. Through the participation of others, they build consensus and commitment around a mission or meaning and a strategy or directions.

There are two primary ways of engaging others in strategic planning: the strategic retreat (see chapter 9) and a formal planning process. Although the two ways can be conceived as independent processes and are often carried out as two separate activities, in reality they are closely linked. A retreat sets the stage for future planning activities by supplying a basic direction that shapes and supports a formal planning effort.

A formal planning effort is a disciplined process, usually carried out on a calendar basis, that requires regularly scheduled discussions on a variety of interrelated supporting elements and decisions. It necessarily involves broad participation of medical staff leaders, middle managers, department heads, and other knowledgeable persons who are convened to test the reality of the strategy, enrich it, and translate it into planned actions. By its very nature, a formal planning system encompasses every level of the organization and feeds on detailed information about operational matters. For these reasons, planning is essentially a bottom-up, broadly participative, cyclical effort that ensures that those expected to carry out the desired actions understand what is expected of them and are able to contribute to developing the plans. In these respects, planning is very different from strategy.

CEOs can choose among varying roles in strategic planning. They can work at the level of thought most appropriate to the situation: *mission,* if the institution lacks shared values; *strategy,* if a framework is needed for making program choices; and *operational planning,* if mission and strategy are in order and capable of shaping future actions. And, of course, CEOs also have a final choice: they can forget about missions, strategies, and plans if things are going well and nothing is changing; they can make tough strategic and planning decisions alone, if this is their preferred style of managing; or they can involve others in creating desired change. CEOs who elect this latter course will find that such an interactive process is both demanding and rewarding and requires that they employ the strategic retreat, a formal planning system, and other appropriate management tools to bring about desired change.

The topics in this chapter can be classified into three different activities: planning, strategy, and step-by-step change (see figure 14, Three Basic Approaches). As the future becomes more uncertain and less subject to an institution's control, hospital leaders must devise an approach to management that fuses all three activities into a meaningful whole. Managers must learn to think in terms of strategic decisions emerging as "continuous, evolving, political, consensus-building processes with no precise beginning or end."[23] They must float trial balloons to determine what is workable, acceptable, or possible. They must be satisfied with partial solutions and be ever wary of making "the best the enemy of the good." None of this may come easy to managers because it calls for new ways of thinking and coping with emerging problems that will affect hospitals and other health care institutions in the future.

This new way of strategic management demands a high level of creative thinking. In managerial terms, creativity is the ability to find new or different ways of looking at or solving problems, to make fundamental changes in the rules to play a new game, to generate many alternatives in a short time, to be willing to consider a wide variety of approaches to a problem, to be alert to little ideas that can lead to big entrepreneurial successes, and to be ready to capitalize on errors, accidents, hunches, and sudden flashes of understanding. These are creative because any one of them can point to ways of doing things differently or better.

But something more is needed. Creativity implies an awareness that there is no one way of doing things, that each organization must develop strategies to fit its own situation. To quote Thomas J. Peters:

"Strategic concepts may be a bit like the rules of the Assassins. That curious medieval sect of Muslim fanatics, we are told, had several orders or ranks, each with its place in an ascending hierarchy. Upon being promoted into the next highest order, initiates would be given a new, and presumably loftier, set of rules to live by. After years during which these strictures became second nature to them, the devout might even find a place in the ninth, or highest order. These few would wait with hushed reverence as the sect's leader welcomed them individually into the elect, whispering into the ear of each the final, ultimate wisdom. The message: 'There are no rules.' "[24]

Yes, there seem to be *no* rules or even one best way of developing strategies for an institution as complex as today's hospital. Each institution must encounter change as it finds it by developing its own sense of mission; by reflecting on its own historic traditions, shared beliefs, managerial values, and community needs; by creating a desired future in terms of some ideal design promoted by its leaders and acceptable to its stakeholder constituencies; and by shaping a workable strategy and plans to enable it to move in a desired direction. Each institution will accomplish these tasks in its own way and in its own time. This book has supplied the reasons to do so and offered some practical advice on how to do it.

Three Basic Approaches

Increasing Uncertainty →

	Long-Range Planning Systems	**Strategy Formulation**	**Step-by-Step Change**
Outside world	Forecastable by extrapolation	Predictable threats and opportunities	Continuously changing flux of urgent issues
Organization emphasis	Bottom-up Staff driven	Top-down Line driven	Mix of staff/line
Characteristics	Multiyear budgets: emphasis on operations, "how" Calendar based	Conceptualization of the business: emphasis on direction, "what"	Messy, learn by doing, loose, flowing, continuous, consensus building process
Key organization variables	Systems (planning)	Strategy and structure	Seven, not two "Soft 5"
Typical approaches	Goals and gaps Comprehensive hospital plan	Total hospital strategy formulation	Emerging issues Stakeholders
Tools	Planning system design	Driving force Portfolio analysis Industry/competitive interaction Trigger for change	Vaguely felt concern Trial balloons Studies Partial solutions Latch on to crises
Key uses	Interface between strategy/tactics creates basis for financial planning	Periodic development of key themes Articulation/conflict Resolution at top	Search for new patterns among emerging strategy of various subsystems (way it is)

Figure 14. All three basic approaches—planning, strategy, and step-by-step change—must be used in effective strategic management.

Notes

1. Bower, Joseph L., and Doz, Yves. Strategy formulation: a social and political process. In: Schendel, Dan E., and Hofer, Charles W., editors. *Strategic Management: A New View of Business Policy and Planning.* Boston: Little, Brown & Company, 1979, p. 154.

2. Ansoff, H. Igor. *Strategic Management.* New York City: John Wiley & Sons, Inc., 1979, p. 128.

3. Weigley, Russell F. *Eisenhower's Lieutenants: The Campaigns of France and Germany 1944-1945.* Bloomington: University of Indiana Press, 1981, p. 286.

4. Saunders Wixen, Joan. Religion at our age. An interview with William Hornaday, Ph.D. In: *Modern Maturity.* 24:27, Aug.-Sept. 1981.

5. For more on the distinction between operational management and strategy, see Schendel, Dan E., and Hofer, Charles W., editors. *Strategic Management: A New View of Business Policy and Planning.* Boston: Little, Brown & Company, 1979, especially chapter 6; Steiner, George A., and Miner, John B. *Management Policy and Strategy.* New York City: Macmillan Publishing Co., Inc., 1977, pp. 7-8; and Ansoff, H. Igor. *Strategic Management.* New York City: John Wiley & Sons, 1979. Nancy Foy observes that the problem of keeping order within an organization and recognizing opportunities to change is a yin-yang situation. It requires "balancing an organization between the tendency to freeze, looking inward, and the tendency to fly apart with all the centrifugal energy—avoiding vicious circles in either direction." Foy, Nancy. *The Yin & Yang of Organizations.* New York City: William Morrow and Company, Inc., 1980, p. 175.

6. Cravens, P. W., and others. *Marketing Decision Making: Concepts and Strategy.* Homewood, IL: Richard D. Irwin, Inc., 1980, p. 90.

7. For more on the concept of environment-serving organizations (organizations whose principal occupation is to supply goods or services to society) see Ansoff.

8. Abell, Derek F., and Hammond, John S. *Strategic Market Planning: Problems and Analyical Approaches.* Englewood Cliffs, NJ: Prentice-Hall, Inc. 1979, p. 63.

9. The American Hospital Association's publications on planning portray this shift in approaches to institutional planning. Its early *Manual on Hospital Planning Procedures,* published in 1959, was intended to be "a comprehensive guide for the planning, organization, and financing involved in almost any type of developmental architectural program." In 1973, the Association published *The Practice of Planning in Health Care Institutions,* which introduced the notion of institutional planning as an ongoing function of management to a wide audience of hospital administrators and trustees, many of whom were "still prone to dismiss planning as a practice useful only to large urban hospitals or to engage in planning only when they contemplate a building program." Two later publications—McMillan, Norman H. *Planning for Survival: A Handbook for Hospital Trustees.* Chicago: AHA, 1978, and Peters, Joseph P. *A Guide to Strategic Planning for Hospitals.* Chicago: AHA, 1979, further attest to what George Stuehler aptly described as AHA's "helping hospital planning to come of age." Simultaneously, the federal government's interest in planning was embodied in section 234 of P.L. 92-603, the Social Security Amendments of 1972, and in various parts of P.L. 93-641, the National Health Planning and Resources Development Act of 1974. More recently, the Joint Commission on Accreditation of Hospitals added a requirement (standard 5) that hospitals establish planning committees with responsibilities for preparing long-range plans to meet community health needs.

10. It is all too easy to fall into the trap of accepting a plan document as the final product of the planning process. One is reminded of the words of Carlos Fuentes, a noted novelist-essayist, who in writing a fictional account of an early Spanish monarch observed, "El Señor had only to consign something to paper and he believed it had an existence of its own; he would not bother again with these minutiae." Fuentes, Carlos. *Terra Nostra.* New York City: Farrar, Straus & Giroux, 1976, p. 158.

11. For more on management's failure to think in strategic terms, see Rothschild, William E. *Putting It All Together: A Guide to Strategic Thinking.* New York City: AMACOM, 1976, pp. 2-4 and chapter 10; also, Don't jump too quickly into goal-setting. *Industry Week.* 180:48, Feb. 11, 1974.

12. See Stuehler, George Jr. A model for planning in health institutions. *Hospital and Health Services Administration.* 23:6, Summer 1978.

13. The authors are indebted to Morris McInnes, Ph.D., senior lecturer, Alfred P. Sloan School of Management, Massachusetts Institute of Technology, Cambridge, for several of the ideas expressed in this and the preceding paragraph.

14. Wildavsky, Aaron. *Speaking Truth to Power: The Art and Craft of Policy Analysis.* Boston: Little, Brown & Company, 1979, p. 9.

15. See, for example, Chandler, Alfred D. Jr. *Strategy and Structure: Chapters in the History of the American*

Industrial Enterprise. Cambridge, MA: MIT Press, 1962; Mintzberg, Henry. *The Structuring of Organizations.* Englewood Cliffs, NJ: Prentice-Hall, Inc., 1979; and Thorelli, Hans B., editor. *Strategy + Structures = Performance: The Strategic Planning Imperative.* Bloomington, IN: University of Indiana Press, 1977.

16. The seven Ss are described in Peters, Thomas J., Organizing for the 80s—farewell to gimmicks . . . back to basics or, keep it simple, stupid. Keynote speech at the Conference-within-the-Conference, The Intersection of Organization Development and Management Consulting—Opportunities for Synergy, Greater Boston OD Network Conference, April 30, 1980. See also Pascale, Richard Tanner, and Athos, Anthony G. *The Art of Japanese Management: Applications for American Executives.* New York City: Simon and Schuster, 1981, and Waterman, R. H. Jr. The seven elements of strategic fit. *Journal of Business Strategy.* 2:69, Winter 1982.

17. Peters, T. J., p. 49.

18. Adapted from Ackoff, Russell L. *Creating the Corporate Future.* New York City: John Wiley & Sons, 1981.

19. Peters, T. J., p. 52.

20. Peters, T. J., p. 51.

21. Mintzberg, Henry. Organization design: fashion or fit? *Harvard Business Review.* 59:103, Jan.-Feb. 1981.

22. An adaptation of some overall conclusions of Allan Kennedy, McKinsey & Company, in a presentation at Boston NASCP, April 4, 1979.

23. Quinn, James Brian. *Strategies for Change: Logical Incrementalism.* Homewood, IL: Richard D. Irwin, Inc., 1980, p. 205.

24. Peters, T. J., p. 54.

Epilogue

This book opened by stating the obvious: hospitals must learn to deal with sudden, often erratic surprises and changes in the outside world that can threaten their survival or affect their activities in unexpected ways. Forecasting future change has never been an easy task; in the present turbulent environment, it has "become a nightmare."[1] Hospital management must now think in terms of rapidly changing conditions, relying not on the carefully formulated long-range master plans of yesterday or on the predict-and-prepare models of more recent vogue, but on developing a sense of direction, a strategy, that enables the institution to survive and thrive in the face of increasing uncertainty.

Much of what was presented in this book was derived from the corporate sector. The literature from this sector continues to present many exciting ideas that can be applied to the art and the practice of strategic planning in hospitals, albeit with care. Hospitals, in turn, are moving rapidly to incorporate some of these ideas on how to deal with their changing environments. With the help of such national groups as the American Hospital Association, hospitals are learning to operate in a political climate radically different from the past, with accompanying changes in Medicare and Medicaid, reduced expenditures for health services, a new federalism, and an emphasis on moving health care more into the mainstream marketplace. Not-for-profit and local government hospitals are also devising ways to deal with severe capital problems. However, as one consultant has observed, "Many of the changes still are not fully appreciated or properly built into the strategic plans and operations of the nation's hospitals."[2]

The point is not whether hospitals are beginning to learn to manage change in uncertain environments, but that so many of them are doing this in new and exciting ways. Corporate restructuring, horizontal and vertical integration, marketing, diversification, corporate separation of some ambulatory care services from the hospital, and new forms of multi-institutional arrangements are no longer alien ideas.[3]

And this is only a beginning. In time, these and other strategies will be widely accepted in the hospital community. Analytical tools from the corporate sector will be increasingly adapted for health care institutions. Planners will become less paper-oriented and more people-oriented as group process skills become paramount in the planning process. As managers come to understand the crucial roles that their institutional values and ambitions play in the process, hospitals will rely less on consultants. Cooperative planning among hospitals that are not already associated with each other in some way will remain spotty, because competition in its many forms will continue to develop and because many areas lack community-based business leaders to promote such cooperation. Planning for multihospital systems will become more and more like corporate planning in decentralized companies and will grow in sophistication.

The next concept on the continuum is strategic management, which is already beginning to be employed by some persons in the health care field. In perhaps three to five years, hospital leaders will increasingly become disillusioned with the concept of strategy predicated on the ability to predict trends and to prepare for them.

Uncertainty, the impact of change, and complexity will exhaust planners' toolkits and frustrate strategists' attempts to control the destinies of their hospitals. Management will then turn to a variety of approaches to managing change, some of which were discussed in this book. Other approaches are emerging from successful experiences in both the corporate and health care sectors.[4] Hospital management must be alert to new ideas, both in terms of process and content, so that they can recharge the capabilities of institutions to deal successfully with change. Indeed, the future promises to be exciting and challenging to those who are willing to meet it on its own terms.

Notes

1. Dixon, Frederick T. Reaganomics, the business cycle, and planning. *Planning Review*. 10:7, July 1982.

2. Brown, Montague. From the editor. *HCM Review*. 7:5, Spring 1982.

3. For more on these and other subjects, see Goldsmith, Jeff C. The health care market: Can hospitals survive? *Harvard Business Review.* Sept.-Oct. 1980.

4. Three recent approaches to strategic planning are summarized in Webber, James B. Ideas outpace reality of hospital strategic planning, but do they pinpoint the future? *Hospitals.* 56:68, Apr. 1, 1982.